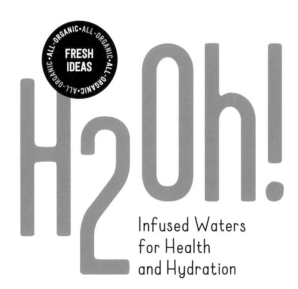

FRESH
IDEAS
·ALL-ORGANIC·ALL-ORGANIC·ALL-ORGANIC·ALL-ORGANIC·ALL-ORGANIC·

H₂Oh!

Infused Waters
for Health
and Hydration

ALSO BY MIMI KIRK

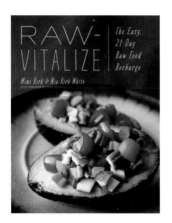 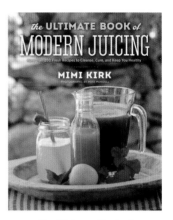

Raw-Vitalize

The Ultimate Book of Modern Juicing

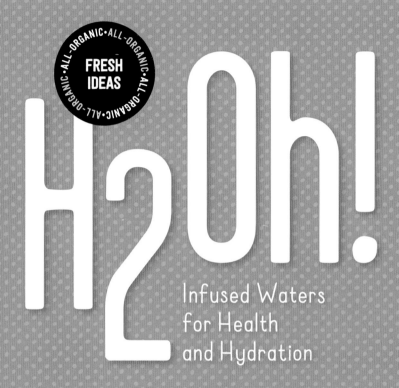

ALL-ORGANIC · ALL-ORGANIC · ALL-ORGANIC · ALL-ORGANIC · ALL-ORGANIC

FRESH IDEAS

H2Oh!

Infused Waters for Health and Hydration

MIMI KIRK

Photographs by Victoria Dodge

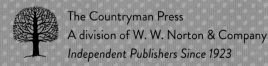

The Countryman Press
A division of W. W. Norton & Company
Independent Publishers Since 1923

All photographs by Victoria Dodge, except for the following:
page v: © bonchan/iStockPhoto.com; vi: © SStajic/iStockPhoto.com; 5: © sirichai_asawalapsakul/iStockPhoto.com; 11: © eskymaks/iStockPhoto.com; 12: ©SergeyPlyusnin/iStockPhoto.com; page 14: © 279photo/iStockPhoto.com; page 17: © Manuta/iStockPhoto.com; 18: © Xanya69/iStockPhoto.com; 21: © ChamilleWhite/iStockPhoto.com; 25: © OlgaMiltsova/iStockPhoto.com; 36: © anna1311/iStockPhoto.com; 40: © natrot/iStockPhoto.com; 44, 99: © Roman Samokhin/iStockPhoto.com; 68: © pioneer111/iStockPhoto.com; 70: ©undefined undefined/iStockPhoto.com; 76 © Besjunior/iStockPhoto.com; 82: © Volosina/iStockPhoto.com; 98: © YuanruLi/iStockPhoto.com.

For information about permission to reproduce selections from this book, write to Permissions, The Countryman Press, 500 Fifth Avenue, New York, NY 10110

For information about special discounts for bulk purchases, please contact W. W. Norton Special Sales at specialsales@wwnorton.com or 800-233-4830

Manufacturing by Versa Press
Book design by Lidija Tomas
Production manager: Devon Zahn

The Countryman Press
www.countrymanpress.com

A division of W. W. Norton & Company, Inc.
500 Fifth Avenue, New York, NY 10110
www.wwnorton.com

978-1-68268-281-4

10 9 8 7 6 5 4 3 2 1

CONTENTS

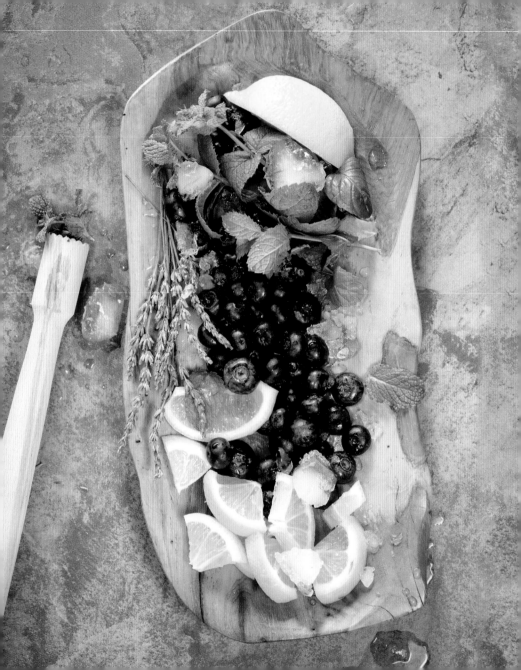

INTRODUCTION

There are few things we need to survive in this world: food, water, air, and of course, our smartphone! In this book we are going to concentrate on water, since there would be neither you nor me nor life on Earth without water.

Water is called by many names in other languages, including:

Spanish—agua
Germain—Wasser
French—eau
Czech—voda

Swedish—vatten
Italian—acqua
Romanian—apă
Islandic—vatn

But in any language—in any country—water is essential for life on this planet.

I'm excited to bring you this book because I've been a water nerd for many years. I was making infused water for my children in the 1970s. Infused water makes me happy, as it's bright and cheerful looking, and it entices me to drink more water, which keeps me healthy.

I became fascinated with water when a friend gave me a book by Masaru Emoto called *The Miracle of Water*. Emoto photographed thousands of water crystals throughout his years of research, proving water absorbs energy and holds memory. The world is made of water, the depth of our oceans is vast, and much of it is still being discovered. If you want to find out more about water energy, you can check out Emoto's book or several YouTube videos on the subject.

Why We Need to Drink Water

Water is working for our body all the time. It rejuvenates and rehydrates us. It aids digestion, flushes out bacteria, and carries nutrients to our cells. It can stabilize our heartbeat and normalize our blood pressure. Water protects our organs and tissues and maintains our electrolyte balance. Hydrated skin starts from the inside. Water plumps up our skin while detoxifying our body. A hydrated body helps keep us looking and feeling younger. Other benefits of drinking infused waters include that they stop sugar cravings and boost metabolism.

Our body is made up of an average of 60 percent water, yet many people do not drink a sufficient amount of it to stay hydrated. Some people say they don't like the taste of water, and some think water has no taste. Others claim water is boring or they can't give up their juice and sugary sodas, but water is proven to be essential to good health. I hope to entice you to drink more water with my infused wet and wild combinations, and that they will replace any sugary drinks you might currently consume.

How Much Water Do We Need to Drink Daily?

Studies have shown somewhere between six and eight glasses a day should be sufficient for most people, but the amount really depends on your health, activity level, and where you live. Warmer climates require drinking more water. We naturally lose water every day through perspiration, urine, and normal bodily functions. We must replenish this loss by the liquids and foods we consume. Sometimes we feel hungry when water is actually all we need. If you feel weak, dizzy, or confused, you might be dehydrated. If you take medication for certain health conditions, consult your doctor regarding how much water you need daily.

Water is the building block of our cells. It helps insulate and regulate our body temperature. Water is needed to metabolize protein and carbohydrates used as food. Water aids digestion. It's our source of saliva and lubricates our joints. Water acts as a shock absorber for our brain, spinal cord, and organs. Water helps flush waste and toxins from our body. Listen to your body and recognize when water is needed. Whatever specific needs your body has, this book will make consuming that quantity easier and more enjoyable.

What Is Infused Water?

in-fuse /in ˈfyooz/

By definition, an infusion is a drink made by placing fruits, herbs, vegetables, or flavorings into a liquid and letting them permeate the liquid for 4 or more hours. Why would we infuse water with herbs and botanicals since water is so perfect in its own right? Well, sipping on the same old thing can get boring, so why not add other beneficial ingredients that might enhance the taste and potency of the water? If you are looking for a way to consume more H_2O, then infusion might be the answer.

Infusion is not only about taste. Potentially, nutrients from the ingredients used to flavor the water can seep in during the process, but to get the full nutritional benefits from produce, you should actually consume the fruit or vegetable as well. In the end, though, the main beneficial ingredient is the water itself and the hydration it provides for maximum health.

How Much Does Infused Water Cost?

Water is the base of all my infusions. You can pay upward of $5 for an 8- to 10-ounce bottle of infused water in your supermarket or convenience store. Store-bought infused waters can be expensive as well as unhealthy. Often they are sugar laden or contain unhealthy sugar substitutes. Many are pasteurized and may contain preservatives. *H2Oh!* provides you with inexpensive, healthy, hydrating recipes that take just minutes to prepare. With the use of organic non-GMO ingredients, filtered water, fruits, vegetables, and herbs, you can enjoy delicious no-calorie drinks at a fraction of the cost of the store-bought variety.

What You Will Find in This Book

In *H2Oh!* you will find delicious combinations of herbs and botanicals to help keep your body hydrated. Being hydrated can improve your health, help with weight loss, encourage energy and vitality, and protect against illness as it flushes out toxins. Infused water makes the act of drinking water more enjoyable, so you are likely to drink more water. The bonus is these infusions have no calories or added sugar and taste delicious.

H2Oh! contains 62 recipes and covers a variety of botanical and medicinal infused waters. You will learn how to make infused ice cubes, which can brighten up your party water with herbs and edible flowers. You can use your infused water and ice cubes for cocktails if you choose to enhance your water intake in this way. Stunning infused water photographs will entice you to crave water over other drinks.

I think you will be delighted with the recipes and knowledge you will gain from *H2Oh!*, as you will start to notice how much better you feel when you are properly hydrated. You will start craving water instead of unhealthy, sugary drinks. These all-natural infused waters will help you detoxify, keep you from eating junk food, improve your mood, clear and plump up your skin, release fat from your cells, help with food digestion and elimination, boost metabolism, control boating, protect against aging, and control false hunger. There's no other drink that compares with the benefits of deliciously infused water!

I hope this makes you thirsty for more!

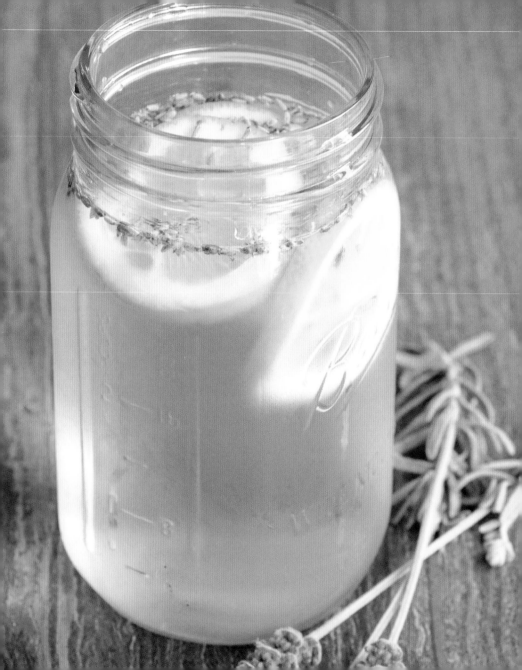

GENERAL INFORMATION

Fruit-infused water is not sweet like fruit juice or smoothies, so expect your infused water to have a light, flavorful taste. Infused waters are refreshing and will keep you away from sugary drinks. Many fruits used in infusions are seasonal, so take advantage when these organic fruits are in season. Fruits contain natural sugars that most bodies can process easily. Frozen fruits can be used as well as fresh fruits, and organic frozen fruit is frozen at peak ripeness, so many times the fruit is even sweeter than fresh. Frozen fruit acts like ice cubes and can chill a drink quickly. Just a reminder, vitamins are in the fruit itself, so be sure to consume the fruit itself after or during infusion.

Some people like to strain the fruit and herbs from the water after chilling for 4 to 24 hours or before drinking. That is a personal preference. Try both ways, removing the infusion or leaving it in as you drink. This way you can decide for yourself which you prefer.

Sweeteners

I do not add sweeteners to my waters, but if you are transitioning from sugary drinks and feel you need a little sweetener, use a dash of pure maple syrup or stevia, never white sugar or chemical sugar substitutes. However, I highly recommend you get used to infused waters without sweeteners. In a few days you will be on board without any sweetener additions.

Vitamin Water

Turn your infused water into vitamin water by adding powders, such as vitamin C or glutamine. These products can be found in health food stores or online. Vitamin C powder is water soluble and known for playing a vital role in building our immune system. It is a highly effective antioxidant, which protects the body's cells from damage by free radicals. Glutamine is an abundant amino acid and plays an important role in muscle protein development. It's a good addition to infused waters after a workout. If you use a liquid vitamin D, you can drop some into any infused water. Be sure to use any of these extra ingredients as the manufacturer directs on the container. Other additions can be kefir water, kombucha, coconut water, or a pinch of Himalayan crystal salt. When including vitamins in your drink, pour the infused water into a glass, add the vitamins, and stir until dissolved.

Equipment Needed

Infused waters need little equipment while providing us with enormous benefits. Here's what you will need:

- Clean glass jars with a tight-fitting lid. Most recipes are based on a 32-ounce (1-quart) mason jar.
- Filtered water
- Ice cube trays
- Fruit, vegetables, and herbs
- Sharp knife and cutting board
- Melon baller (optional)
- Muddler or wooden spoon for crushing fruit and herbs

What You Should Know Before You Start

- Fruit, vegetables, and herbs should be organic whenever possible. Wash all produce and rinse herbs. Peel anything that is not organic.

- Drink infused water within 24 to 48 hours, or strain the solid ingredients from the water if keeping for a longer time. Each infusion is different and all fruits respond differently, so tasting is your best judge of freshness. With the infused solids removed, water will be good for another day or two.

- Eat any infused fruit whenever possible, anywhere from 4 to 24 hours after infusing. Keep in mind that eating the fruit or vegetable ensures you get its full nutritional value.

- Remove the rind and white pith from orange, lime, grapefruit, and lemon after 4 hours of infusing, as the rind starts to bitter the water. If you remove the rind after 4 hours, the fruit can go back into the water for a longer period of time.

- Crush herbs by rubbing them between your fingers or palms, or use a wooden spoon or muddler to activate the oils in the herbs.

- The quality of your water is important. Use room-temperature or cold filtered or purified water for fruit and vegetable infusions.

- Use your own taste buds to determine when and whether you want to remove an infused fruit, vegetable, or herb. Some of these ingredients work quicker than others, and although they look good in the jar, the idea is to flavor the water. As you drink throughout the day, you can always add more water to the infusion as well, or remove the solid contents and continue to drink the infused water.

- Ice cubes can be added to any infusion. Put ice cubes in a glass and pour in the infusion.

- Always use filtered water to make ice cubes.

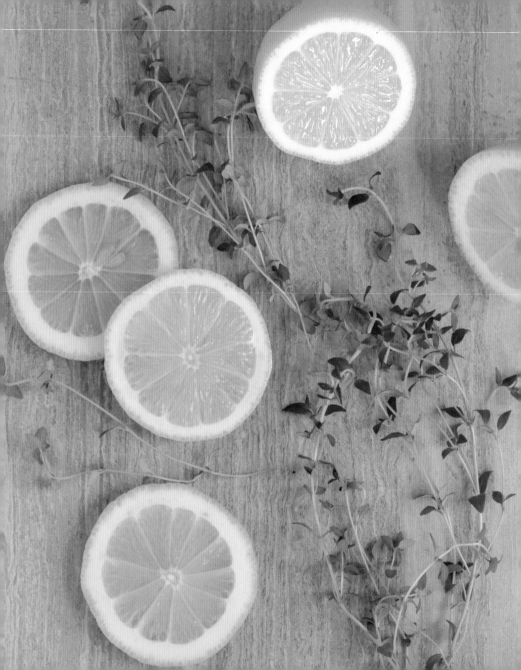

TAKE THE WATER CHALLENGE

Try this challenge: drink eight 8-ounce glasses of infused water per day for 21 days. In this short length of time you will start craving infused waters, you will create a new habit, and you will look and feel better. Before you start the 21 days, notice whether you have bags or dark circles under your eyes. Notice whether you are tired in the afternoon or have brain fog. Notice how your body feels when you wake up in the morning. When you complete the 21 days, notice whether there is any change in the bags or dark circles.

- Have they lightened or disappeared?

- Has your skin improved?

- Has your energy and aliveness shown a noticeable change?

Trying this challenge will help you become a lifelong fan of infused water. Even more fun is to do it with a friend or a group of friends, and enjoy the results of helping others stay hydrated and feel the effects of infused water.

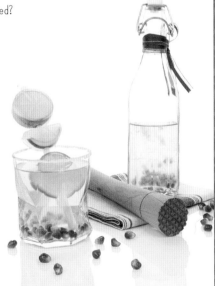

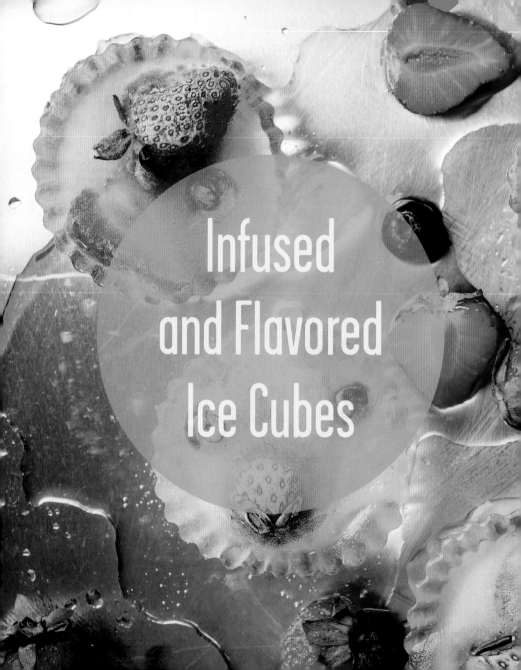

Infused
and Flavored
Ice Cubes

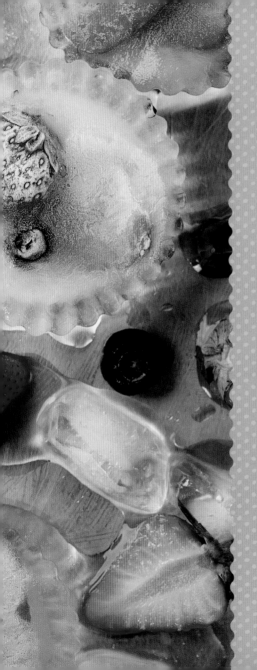

The plain clear or frosted ice cube can now show signs of beauty as an addition to any drink. Water is a great thirst quencher and healthy on its own, but by tossing some infused ice cubes into a favorite pretty glass, you have created an exciting summer delight. Infused or flavored ice cubes are perfect for sparkling water, mocktails, cocktails, or infused waters.

Infused ice cubes are simple to make, and you can find many ice trays in different shapes and sizes online or in kitchen stores. The newer flexible rubber molds make removing the cubes easy. Some of these rubber cube trays are for chocolate making but work for ice cubes as well. The nice thing about rubber molds is you don't have to run water on them to get the cubes out. The older models of ice cube trays are not as easy to remove the cube. It's well worth the investment to buy the new molds for the years of pleasure they will bring.

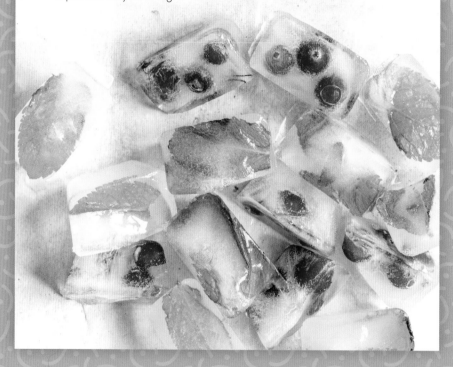

How to Make Infused Ice Cubes

1. Prepare all the ingredients you wish to infuse: wash and chop to size.

2. Place the ingredients in the ice cube tray.

3. Fill the tray with filtered water.

4. Freeze until frozen solid.

5. When frozen, remove the cubes from the tray and store in the freezer in resealable plastic bags or a glass container.

TIP 1:

If you lightly boil your filtered water once or twice and let it cool down before pouring into your ice cube trays, it helps keep the frozen cubes clear and not cloudy. Lightly boiled water means not to a full rolling boil. Turn off the heat just before the water comes to a full boil and let it cool down.

TIP 2:

Work quickly when removing ice cubes from their tray and bagging them to be sure the cubes don't melt, or else they might freeze together when storing.

TIP 3:

Try filling the ice cube tray to half its depth with filtered water and freeze until just barely frozen, about 20 minutes. Place fruit or an herb on top of each shallow cube and fill the rest of the way with additional water. This gives a different effect to the frozen cube. You can leave a little piece of herb or fruit sticking out for a fun look.

HERE ARE SOME OF MY FAVORITE ICE CUBE COMBINATIONS:

JUST BASIL

No, really, this is an amazing infusion and one of my favorites. Pop a basil leaf into each compartment of an ice cube tray and fill with filtered water. Freeze until solid.

JUST MINT

Just pop a leaf or two into each compartment of an ice cube tray and fill with filtered water. Freeze until solid.

For all the following combinations, just follow directions on How to Make Infused Ice Cubes (page 14):

- Lemonade + Mint + Lemon Zest
- Basil + Watermelon
- Basil + Strawberry
- Mint + Blackberry
- Lime + Blackberry
- Blueberry + Raspberry
- Kiwi + Blueberry

- Lemon + Lime
- Pineapple + Mint
- Cherry with stem sticking out
- Orange + Cranberry
- Cucumber + Mint
- Blueberry + Lemon
- Apple sprinkled with ground cinnamon

EDIBLE FLOWERS

Edible flowers make beautiful infused ice cubes and can be purchased at many health food stores and specialty stores. Ask your produce department if it carries them. Don't use dried or nonedible flowers, or flowers that have been sprayed or grown with pesticides.

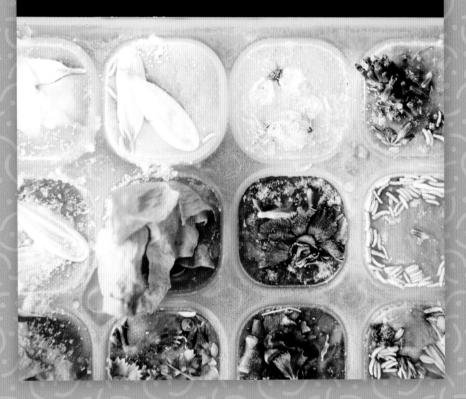

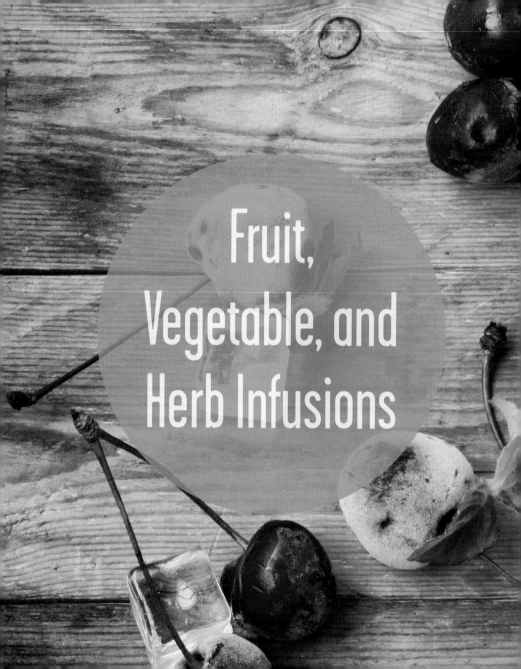

Fruit, Vegetable, and Herb Infusions

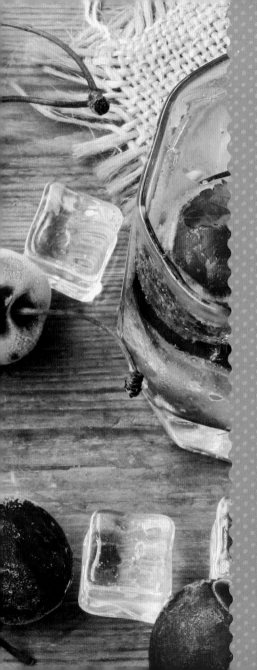

Sipping on infused water all day will make a big difference in your inner and outer body. Keep a jar on your desk and sip every hour. A filled 32-ounce mason jar will give you half of your daily water requirement. Chilled water is great, but don't forget it's in the refrigerator. You are less likely to forget if you have a container right next to you, especially if you're sitting at your desk most of the day.

The way you cut your fruit—thick, thin, halved, or quartered—is all up to you. Since it's good to eat the fruit for total nutritional value, pack your jar with as much fruit as you want. It doesn't take much fruit to infuse the water, but extra fruit will be delicious to snack on.

Some fruits take longer than others to infuse water. Herbs, such as basil or mint, infuse quickly, as do citrus, cucumbers, and melons. Harder ingredients, such as apples, ginger, and cinnamon stick, may take an overnight soak to release their essence into the water. Soft fruits, such as strawberries and watermelon, can get waterlogged quickly; remove soft fruit from the water and eat within 6 hours. Blueberries and cranberries will still be fresh overnight. Removing the rind from citrus fruits at the 4-hour point will keep water from turning bitter, or cut off the rind, including the white pith, before infusing.

Follow the recipes when starting out. Then, when you feel comfortable, create some of your own combinations. This book contains some common fruit infusions, such as apple, orange, and berries, but many infusions go beyond these common fruits to create unique flavors. After tasting hundreds of infused combinations, I found certain flavors work better with some flavors than others, which allowed me to bring the best combinations to *H2Oh!* The tastier the combination, the more water you will drink, and you will find yourself referring back to the book to keep waters varied, interesting, and delicious.

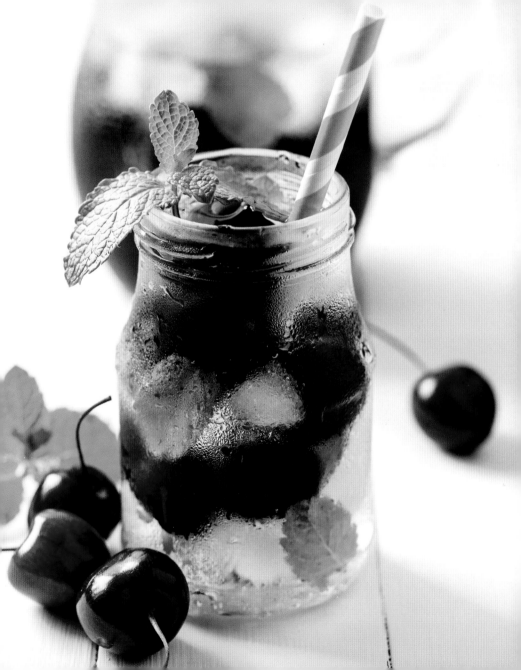

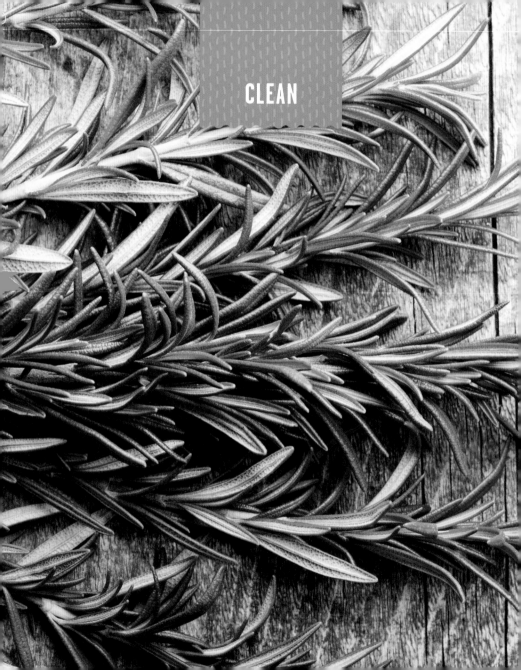

CLEAN

rosemary water

Rosemary can boost memory, improve mood, relieve inflammation, stimulate circulation, detoxify the body from bacteria, and heal skin conditions. Those are good enough reasons to drink rosemary infusions, but my favorite story about the benefits of rosemary is about Queen Elizabeth of Hungary, who suffered from crippling gout and rheumatism. She claimed at the age of 72 that drinking rosemary water helped her regain her beauty and strength. As the story goes, she even received a marriage proposal from the king of Poland—who was 26!

1 sprig rosemary

Filtered water

Place the rosemary in a 32-ounce mason jar, top up with the water, chill, and drink.

apple + cardamom + lemon

Cardamom is a mouth freshener. This might not be important since drinking lots of water helps with stale mouth as well, but the taste of cardamom is delightful. The pods have a hard shell, so just give them a slight crush with your knife before infusing. Apple will provide nutrients when you eat the fruit from the infusion. Lemon is added to kick up the flavor and for alkalizing.

½ apple
5 cardamom pods
2 lemon slices
Filtered water

1. Slice the apple thinly.

2. Crush the cardamom pods with the flat end of your chopping knife, just enough to break the shell slightly.

3. Add the apple slices, pods, and lemon slices to a 32-ounce mason jar and top up with the water.

4. Let chill in the refrigerator for 4 or more hours. Remove the rind and white pith of the lemon after 4 hours to prevent bitterness. You can refill the bottle with more filtered water when you drink half of the infused water. Be sure to eat the apple slices at the end of the day.

basil water

Basil is one of my favorite infusers. Just adding basil alone is enough for me to drink eight glasses of water daily. Dried leaves do not have the same oils as fresh, so using fresh basil leaves for infusing is a must.

5 fresh basil leaves
Filtered water

1. Place the basil in a 32-ounce mason jar, top up with the water, and chill 4 or more hours.

— HEALTH NOTE —

Basil is anti-inflammatory and helpful for rheumatoid arthritis. Basil enhances circulation and stabilizes blood sugar.

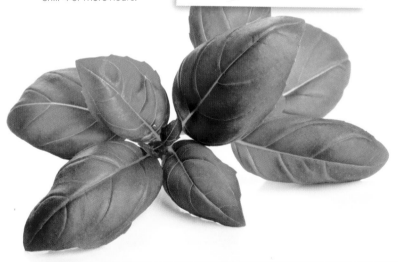

blackberry + mint

Blackberry season is quite short, so be sure to make this infusion during peak time, when berries are the sweetest and at the best price. Blackberries' high antioxidant levels can reduce inflammation. They contain vitamin C and are good for skin. Mint is the perfect blend with blackberry infusion.

12 blackberries
2 fresh mint leaves
Filtered water
Ice cubes (optional)

1. To extract the flavor from the berries, lightly crush them in a 32-ounce mason jar, using a muddler or wooden spoon.

2. Crush the mint leaves between your fingers to extract the essence. Place the leaves in the jar with the berries and top up with the water. Add ice cubes, if desired, or chill for 4 hours in the refrigerator.

3. Scoop out the berries to consume when the water tastes infused to your liking.

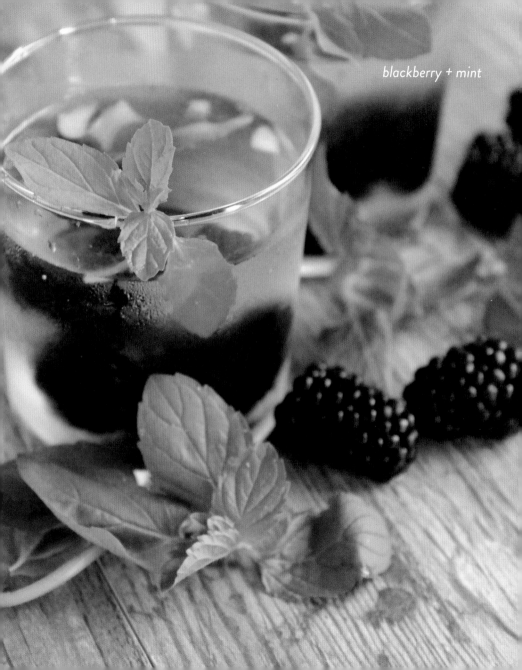

blackberry + mint

cantaloupe + mint + lime

The best time to eat cantaloupes is when the sweet fruit is in peak season. It's also the best time to make this flavorful infusion. The best hydration you can get comes from water, and with infusions like cantaloupe, you will certainly want to drink more.

1 cup peeled, chunked, or sliced cantaloupe
(use a melon baller if you have one)

2 or 3 fresh mint leaves

½ lime, seeded and sliced

Filtered water

1. Place the cantaloupe, mint, and lime slices in a 32-ounce mason jar and top up with the water.

2. Chill for 4 or more hours and eat the melon when the water tastes infused from the fruit. Remove the rind and white pith of the lime after 4 hours to prevent bitterness.

—— HEALTH NOTE ——

Cantaloupe has the highest beta-carotene of any yellow or orange fruit and the same amount as carrots. Once eaten, beta-carotene is converted into vitamin A and acts as a powerful antioxidant that helps fight free radicals. Beta-carotene is good for eye health and healthy blood cells. Cantaloupe contains vitamin C and folate. It's also good for a quick hydration.

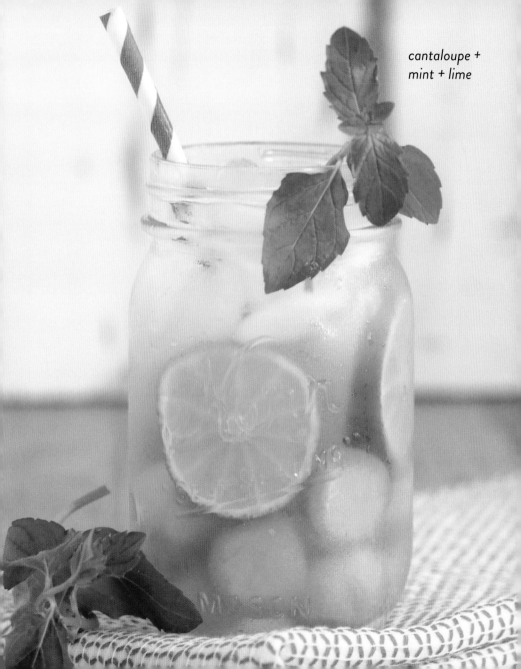

cantaloupe +
mint + lime

cucumber + cilantro

"Simply delicious" is all that can be said about this infusion. The forever flavorful, detoxifying cucumber can be light enough to drink with any meal. It's true, not everyone likes cilantro, but if you're one of the lucky ones who enjoys this herb, you will really love this infusion. Cilantro is an anti-inflammatory herb which also lowers blood sugar. Use parsley if you are not a cilantro lover.

One 2-inch piece cucumber
4 sprigs fresh cilantro, including stems
Filtered water

1. Peel the cucumber, if you desire, or leave the skin on (see note). Slice and place in a 32-ounce mason jar.

2. Add the cilantro and top up with the water.

3. Chill for 4 hours. The cucumber and cilantro can be removed at this time if the infusion is flavored to your liking.

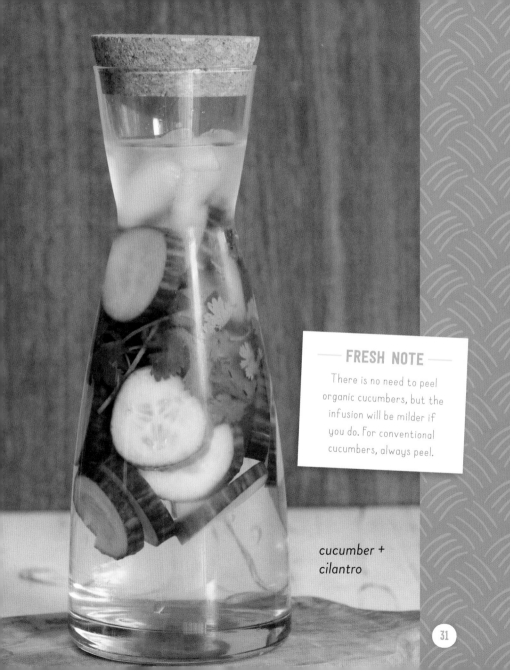

cucumber + cilantro

cucumber + mint

The combinations provided in this book might only have simple changes, but they are made to keep your infusions interesting. If you have a favorite and drink it daily, eventually you will want an alternative. This infusion is a simple change from the citrus-cucumber infusions.

One 2-inch piece cucumber
2 fresh mint leaves
Filtered water

1. Peel the cucumber, if you desire, or leave the skin on (see note on page 31). Slice and place in a 32-ounce mason jar.

2. Crush the mint leaves between your fingers to release their flavor. Add to the jar and top up with the water.

3. Chill for 3 to 4 hours. Remove the cucumber and mint when the desired taste is achieved or add more water to dilute.

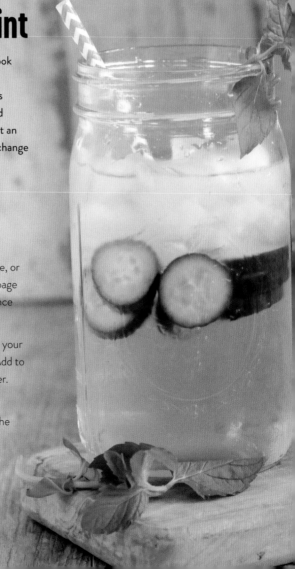

cucumber + mint + lemon

This is only a change in citrus from another infusion, but the taste is quite different. Lemons and limes have the same nutrient value and contain vitamin C. They are from the same citrus family but are different in color. Also lemons are sourer than limes unless you are lucky enough to find the Meyer lemon, which is quite sweet. Lemon or lime, it's up to your taste buds.

One 3-inch piece cucumber

2 fresh mint leaves

2 lemon slices

Filtered water

1. Remove the skin from the cucumber and slice to your liking.

2. Crush the mint leaves to release the flavor.

3. Peel the rind and white pith from the lemon slices.

4. Place the cucumber, mint, and lemon slices in a 32-ounce mason jar and top up with the water.

grapefruit + rosemary

Grapefruit's health benefits are many. Grapefruit is known to contain potassium, lycopene, and vitamins A and C. It's also are very low in calories and good for clear skin. If you are taking medication, check with your doctor, as grapefruit can cause adverse reactions if consumed during certain drug regimens. The pink variety is always sweeter. Choose smooth skin with small pores for the tastiest fruit.

½ to 1 grapefruit
One 1-inch sprig rosemary
Filtered water

1. Wash the grapefruit and slice thickly. If removing the rinds, do so before slicing.

2. Place the sliced grapefruit and rosemary in a 32-ounce mason jar and top up with the water.

3. Chill for 4 or more hours in the refrigerator. Taste for flavor and remove the grapefruit and rosemary when the water is to your liking. If left on, remove the rind and white pith of the fruit after 4 hours to prevent bitterness. Eat the fruit for a healthy snack.

FRESH NOTE

You will find that the rind on citrus fruits starts to bitter the water after a while. Remove the rind and white pith from the grapefruit if you plan to leave the infusion more than 4 hours. You can start out with the rind on and eat the grapefruit as soon as the water is infused. The grapefruit makes a great snack, and you will be sure to obtain all the nutrients from the fruit.

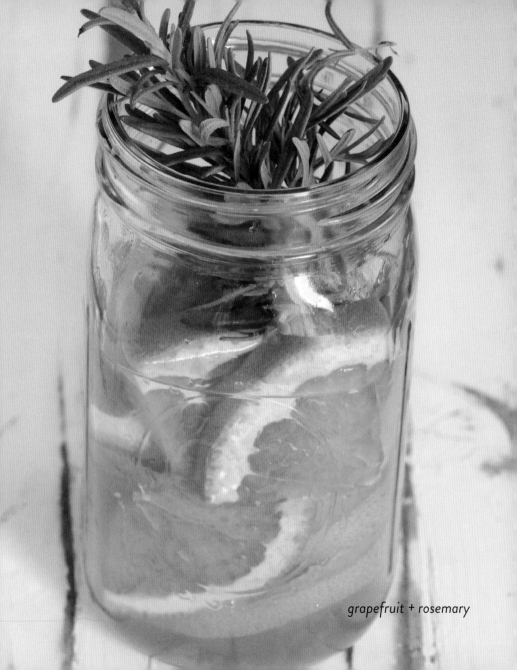

grapefruit + rosemary

grapefruit + lemon + lime + orange

What do citrus fruits have in common? To start, they are high in vitamin C and antioxidants. Except for the kumquat, citrus fruits have thick rinds and juicy pulp. They are a seeded fruit, contain segments, and grow in hot climates. Eat the grapefruit and orange from the infusion for full nutritional value. Squeeze the lemon and lime in the water for a stronger infusion.

½ grapefruit

1 orange

½ lemon

½ lime

Filtered water

1. Slice the grapefruit and orange thickly, and the lemon and lime thinly. If removing the rinds, do so before slicing.

2. Place all the sliced fruits in a 32-ounce mason jar and top up with the water.

3. Chill for 4 or more hours in the refrigerator. Taste for flavor and remove the grapefruit and orange when the water is to your liking. If left on, remove the rind and white pith of the fruit after 4 hours to prevent bitterness. Eat the fruit for a healthy snack.

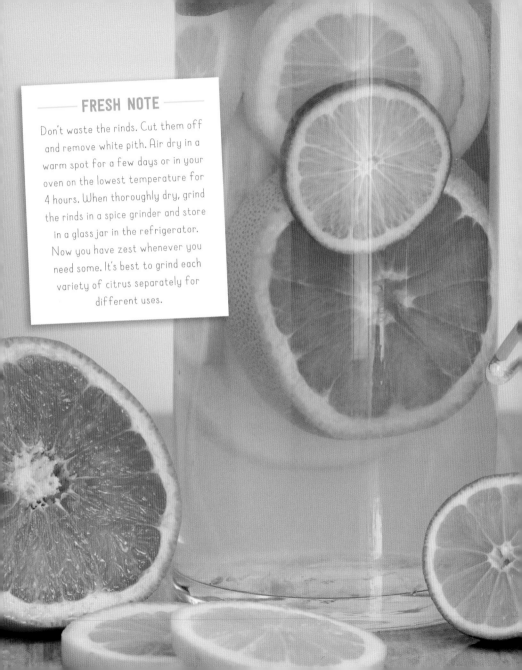

FRESH NOTE

Don't waste the rinds. Cut them off and remove white pith. Air dry in a warm spot for a few days or in your oven on the lowest temperature for 4 hours. When thoroughly dry, grind the rinds in a spice grinder and store in a glass jar in the refrigerator. Now you have zest whenever you need some. It's best to grind each variety of citrus separately for different uses.

grapefruit + pineapple + mint

A pink grapefruit would make a beautiful infusion. Grapefruit can be sweet, tart, or even bitter. Regardless of color or flavor, it packs a combination of potassium, lycopene, vitamins A and C, and choline. It's good for heart health and known for weight loss. Add some pineapple for sweetness, enzymes, and eye and bone heath. Protect your health by eating the fruit and enjoying the water from a tasty infusion.

2 or 3 fresh mint leaves

2 thick grapefruit slices

½ cup pineapple chunks

Filtered water

1. Crush the mint between your fingers to release the oils and for the full essence.

2. Place the mint, grapefruit, and pineapple in a 32-ounce mason jar, top up with the water, and chill in the refrigerator. Remove the rind and white pith of the grapefruit after 4 hours to prevent bitterness.

— FRESH NOTE —

The grapefruit infuses quickly, so you will appreciate the taste even after the grapefruit is removed. (Remove the grapefruit after 4 hours if you leave the rind on or 5 to 6 hours if the rind has been removed.) The pineapple and mint can stay in the container, but be sure to eat the pineapple as well to get all the nutrition.

lemon + basil

The taste of lemon and stress-reducing basil makes a very light and refreshing infusion. Basil is also good for detoxifying the liver. It's easy to drink and takes seconds to prepare. You will find a recipe for basil-infused ice cubes on page 16.

2 large fresh basil leaves

3 or 4 lemon slices

Filtered water

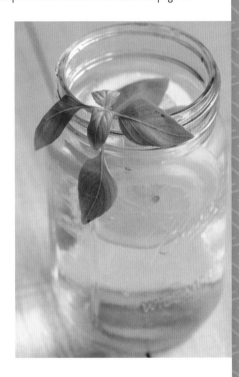

1. Crush the basil lightly with your fingers to activate the essential oils.

2. Place the basil and lemon slices in a 32-ounce mason jar and top up with the water.

3. Refrigerate for 4 hours or overnight. Remove the rind and white pith of the lemon after 4 hours to prevent bitterness.

lemon + crushed ginger

From previous descriptions you know the alkalizing effects of lemon, but did you know ginger helps with inflammation? Ginger is a powerful medicinal root. Ginger can help in digestion and fighting colds. It can stop nausea and reduce the risk of heart disease. To get the full benefits, ginger should be crushed or made into a tea (see note, right).

One 1-piece piece fresh ginger

1 lemon

Filtered water

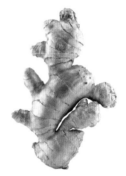

1. Use a knife or the edge of a teaspoon to scrape the skin off the ginger. To crush the ginger, make small cuts in the ginger, then lay it flat on a chopping board. With a large chopping knife, lay the flat, thicker part of the knife on top of the ginger. Smash your fist on top of the flattened part of the knife. Pound several times until the ginger is broken up.

2. Remove the rind and white pith from the lemon and slice.

3. Place the ginger and lemon slices in a 32-ounce mason jar, top up with the water, and chill.

H2Oh! · Infused Waters for Health and Hydration

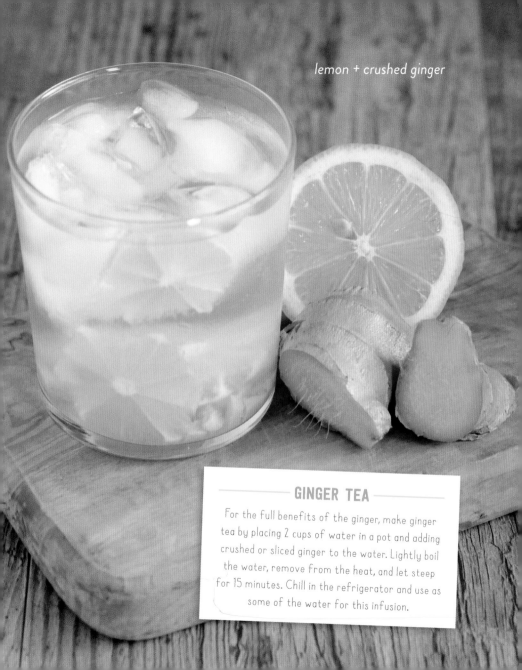

lemon + crushed ginger

GINGER TEA

For the full benefits of the ginger, make ginger tea by placing 2 cups of water in a pot and adding crushed or sliced ginger to the water. Lightly boil the water, remove from the heat, and let steep for 15 minutes. Chill in the refrigerator and use as some of the water for this infusion.

lemon + crushed ginger + mint

Mint is a cleanser for the blood and a digestive agent as well. Add alkalizing lemon and crushed ginger for anti-inflammatory affects and you will enjoy a powerful infusion.

3 or 4 lemon slices

One 1-inch piece ginger

3 fresh mint leaves

Filtered water

— FRESH NOTE —

Use ginger tea (page 41) for part or all of water.

1. Peel away the rind and white pith of the lemon slices, or leave on.

2. Use a knife or the edge of a teaspoon to scrape the skin off the ginger. To crush the ginger, make small cuts in the ginger, then lay it flat on a chopping board. With a large chopping knife, lay the flat, thicker part of the knife on top of the ginger. Smash your fist on top of the flattened part of the knife. Pound several times until the ginger is broken up.

3. Place the lemon slices and ginger in a 32-ounce mason jar and top up with the water. If left on, remove the rind and white pith of the lemon after 4 hours to prevent bitterness.

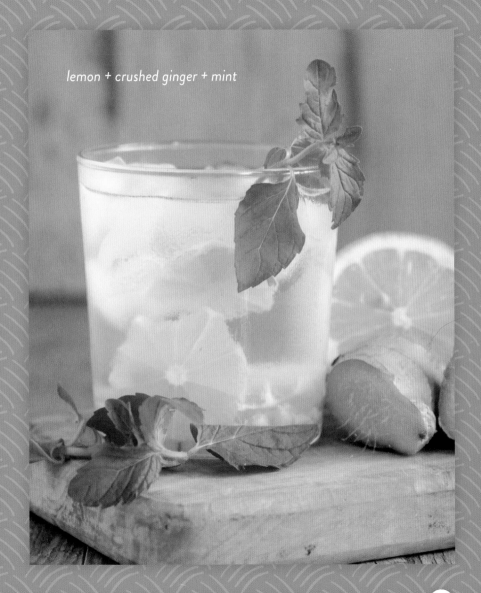

lemon + crushed ginger + mint

lemon

Lemon and water is a great detoxifier. Having a glass in the morning on an empty stomach helps alkalinize the body. Sipping lemon water daily can be beneficial for the immune system and digestion.

½ lemon

Filtered water, at room temperature

Squeeze the juice from the half lemon into an 8-ounce glass of the water.

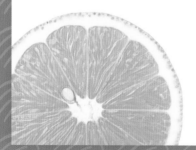

lemon + mint

The combination of lemon and mint go hand in hand for a perfect detoxifying balance.

1 lemon

3 or 4 mint leaves, or a small sprig

Filtered water

1. Slice the lemon, peel away the rind and white pith of the slices, or leave on.

2. Place the lemon slices and mint in a 32-ounce mason jar and top up with the water.

3. Mint infuses water quickly, so take a sip and remove the mint when the flavor suits your taste.

4. When the water is half gone, add more to fill the jar.

5. If left on, remove the rind and white pith of the lemon after 4 hours so as not to bitter the water.

lemon + lime + thyme

This combination will be a unique way to drink more water. We know the alkalizing value of lemon, and the taste of lime is sure to brighten your water. Lime contains calcium and folate, and thyme is a great source of iron and a powerful anti-inflammatory.

3 lemon slices

3 lime slices

1 sprig thyme

Filtered water

1. Place the lemon and lime slices in a 32-ounce mason jar.

2. Pinch the thyme leaves to release the oils and place them in the jar.

3. Top up with the water and chill, if desired.

4. Remove the rind and white pith of the lemon and lime after 4 hours to prevent bitterness.

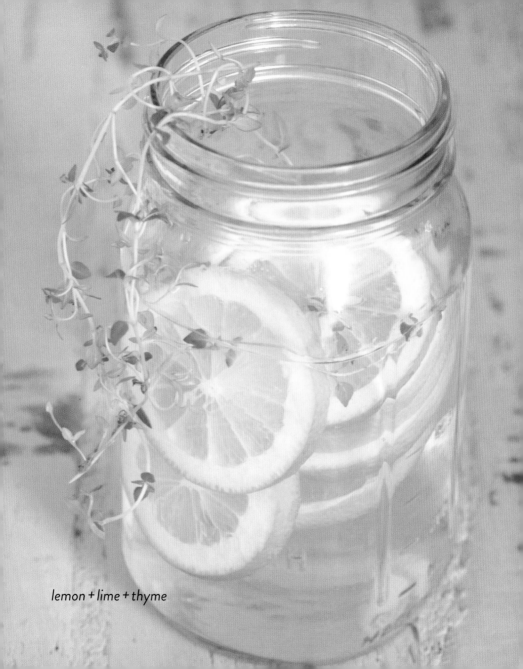

lemon + lime + thyme

lemon + strawberries = pink lemonade

Strawberries make a beautiful, enticing infusion. The properties in strawberries can help burn stored fat and can lower the risk of heart disease. Eat the strawberries to obtain all their nutritional value.

4 or 5 strawberries

1 lemon

Filtered water

1. Muddle or crush the strawberries lightly with a wooden spoon. This will extract flavor into the water.

2. Remove the rind and white pith of the lemon or leave on to infuse.

3. Place the strawberries and lemon slices in a 32-ounce mason jar and top up with the water. Alternatively, place the strawberries and a scant

4 cups of water in a blender and blitz, pour into a 32-ounce mason jar, and add the lemon slices.

4. If left on, remove the rind and white pith of the lemon after 4 hours to prevent bitterness. Nice when chilled.

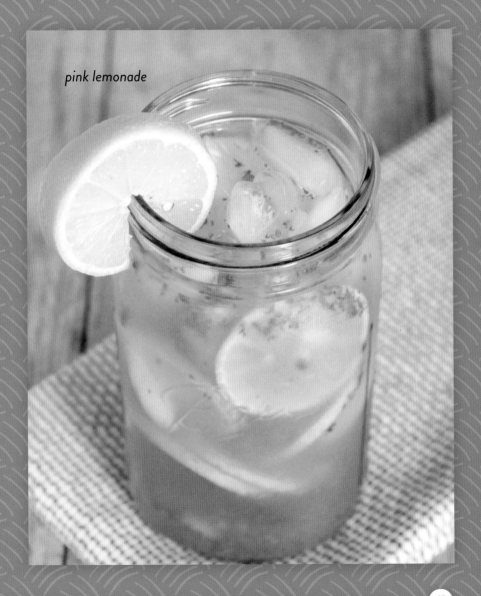

pink lemonade

strawberry + mint

Just can't get enough of strawberries when they are in season, right? Well, I know I can't. Organic strawberries are so sweet and satisfying as a snack, so why not have them in water with some mint and eat them when the water is infused? Hydration and a snack are always good.

6 strawberries

1 small sprig mint

Filtered water

1. Wash the strawberries and cut in half.

2. Place the strawberries and mint sprig in a 32-ounce mason jar, top up with the water, and chill.

3. Enjoy eating the strawberries throughout the day.

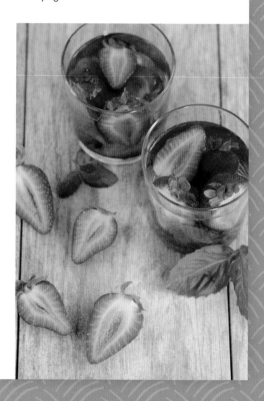

peach + mint

The taste of a summer peach lingers in your mind long after they are gone from the market. They ripen very quickly and go bad before you know it, so slice some up, line a baking sheet with parchment paper, and freeze the slices. When frozen, place in a glass container or resealable plastic bag. Freeze a sprig of mint along with the peaches and you are ready for some delicious infused water.

2 peaches
1 sprig mint
Filtered water

1. Wash, slice, and pit the peaches.

2. Place the peach slices and mint in a 32-ounce mason jar and top up with the water.

3. Chill for 5 or more hours.

── HEALTH NOTE ──

Peaches offer a rich array of potassium, calcium, iron, magnesium, manganese, zinc, and copper.

orange + mint

In parts of the world, oranges are abundant; in other areas, they are seasonal. In season is the ideal time to make orange infusions. Orange infusions can also be made with a splash of orange juice as well. You will still get some nutritional value and it may lift your spirits during cold weather. Add the mint to aid digestion.

1 orange
2 or 3 fresh mint leaves
Filtered water

1. Wash the orange and thickly slice.

2. Crush the mint leaves in your fingers to release their essence.

3. Place the orange slices and mint in a 32-ounce mason jar and top up with the filtered water.

4. Crush a little of the orange into the water, using a muddler or wooden spoon.

5. Infuse in the refrigerator for 4 or more hours. Remove the rind and white pith of the orange after 4 hours to prevent bitterness.

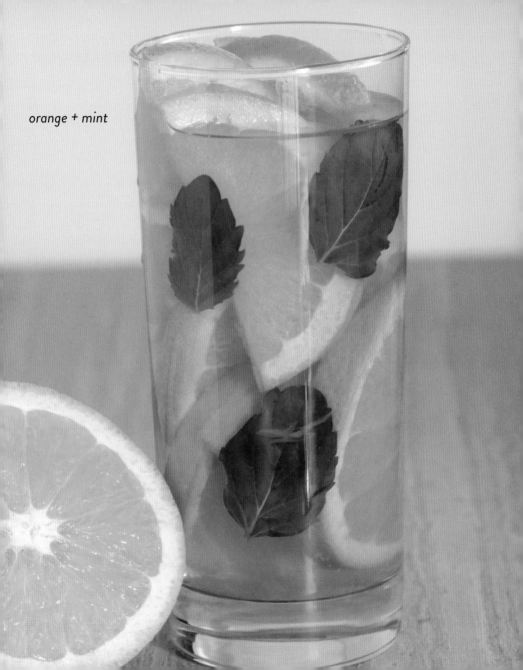

orange + mint

strawberry + thyme

Make thyme tea and let it cool to use as the water for this infusion. In this way, you will get the best extract from the thyme. Consuming the strawberries will give you all their nutrients as well as flavor the tea water.

3 spigs fresh thyme or 2 teaspoons dried thyme

Filtered water

5 or 6 strawberries

1. Make thyme tea the night before making this infusion by gently boiling fresh or dried thyme in 4 cups of the water. Let steep for about 10 minutes and strain. Chill overnight or for at least 4 hours.

2. Wash and hull the strawberries and cut in half.

3. Place in a 32-ounce mason jar and top up with the chilled thyme tea. The strawberries should infuse in about 4 hours. Don't forget to eat the strawberries.

— HEALTH NOTE —

Thyme is an antibacterial an anti-inflammatory herb.

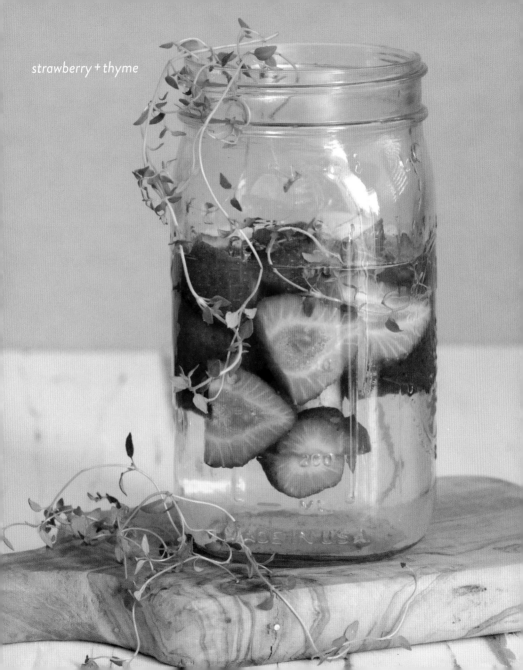

strawberry + thyme

strawberry + basil

Sweet strawberries and mild basil make a perfect match. This water goes with any meal and is delicious after a workout. Eat the strawberries as soon as the water is infused to your liking. Strawberries' anthocyanins help burn stored fat and lower the risk of heart disease, so eat your strawberries and enjoy the infused water.

5 or 6 strawberries
2 fresh basil leaves
Filtered water

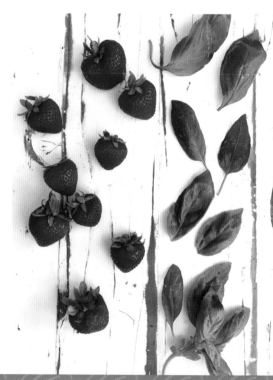

1. Wash and hull the strawberries and slice in half.

2. Crush the basil between your fingers.

3. Place the strawberries and basil in a 32-ounce mason jar, top up with the water, and chill for 4 hours.

watermelon + mint

Nothing says "summer" like watermelon, and summer is a perfect time to consume more water. Watermelon is 92 percent water. Add a little mint and you have a thirst-quenching drink.

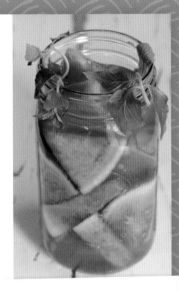

As many small wedges of
   watermelon as you like

2 or 3 fresh mint leaves

Filtered water

1. Place a couple of wedges of watermelon and mint in a 32-ounce mason jar. Press the ingredients with a wooden spoon or muddler to release the flavor.

2. Add a few more watermelon wedges, then top up the jar with the water. Chill in refrigerator for 4 hours.

3. Strain the melon from the water before drinking (see note).

—— FRESH NOTE ——

Eat the ice-cold watermelon from your water for vitamin C. It's a good source of beta-carotene and lycopene, and it's anti-inflammatory, too. Agua fresca is a water-based drink typical in Mexico. A variety of fruits are used. To make Watermelon Agua Fresca, place all the above ingredients in a blender and blitz. Serve over ice.

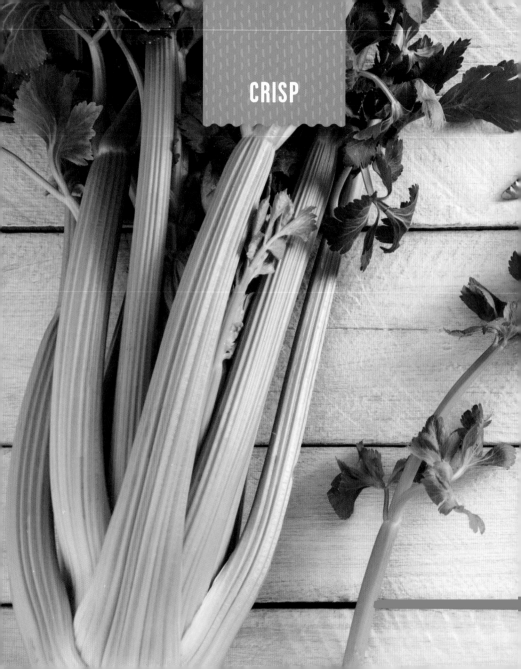

CRISP

cucumber + celery

The taste of infused cucumber is great, very refreshing, and always good after a workout. Cucumber is good for digestion and detoxifying, so be sure to eat the cucumber. Cucumber picks up the infusion flavor quickly. Celery adds a wonderful taste with a little salty flavor. This combination could end up being one of your favorites.

One 2-inch piece cucumber
1 celery rib
Filtered water

1. Peel the cucumber and slice to your desired thickness.

2. Cut the celery into three pieces.

3. Place the cucumber and celery in a 32-ounce mason jar and top up with the water. Chill until the flavors are combined.

apple + ginger

Antioxidants help reduce the risk of cancer, hypertension, heart disease, and diabetes, all good reasons to eat apples. Apples are a good source of B-complex vitamins and dietary fiber as well. Be sure to slice up enough apples, as they infuse slowly. You can snack on the apples all day, as they hold up well in infusions. Ginger is known to be an anti-inflammatory and can help cleanse the walls of your intestines and liver, so it's a good detoxifier and immunity booster.

1 or 2 apples

One 1-inch piece fresh ginger (see note)

Filtered water

1. Thinly slice the apples, removing the seeds and stem.

2. Crush or slice the ginger thinly or substitute ginger tea (see note).

3. Place the apples and ginger in a 32-ounce mason jar, top up with the water, and chill. Nice served over ice

FRESH NOTE

Slicing freshly peeled ginger into room temperature water is fine if you are just looking for a light infusion. Alternatively, to get the most from your ginger, make fresh ginger tea by lightly boiling a 1-inch piece of peeled, sliced ginger in 4 cups of filtered water. You can cool down the tea in the refrigerator and add the apple slices right to the cooled tea. Extracting the ginger in a tea makes a stronger infusion.

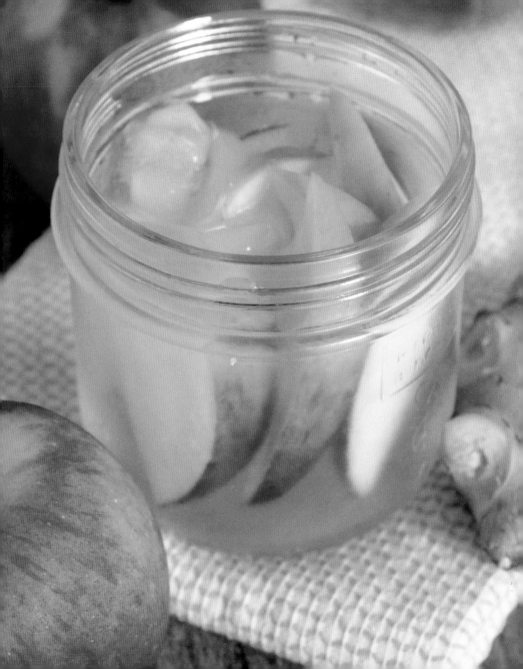

apple + cranberry + mango + rosemary

We are getting dangerously creative with this combination. Cranberries might be difficult to find year-round, but check the frozen food department. When they are in season, purchase extra and freeze for a later date. Cranberries need a little crush. Just place them on a cutting board and place the flat of your knife on top. Give a light pound with your fist, just enough to burst open or crush the berry. This will help strengthen the infusion. Mango has a sweeter flavor and helps with a variety of health issues. Mango lowers cholesterol, alkalizes the body, improves digestion, and helps fight heatstroke. With a hint of rosemary and apple, this drink will satisfy your thirst and make you feel good all over.

½ apple

⅓ cup cranberries

¼ mango

One 1-inch sprig rosemary

Filtered water

1. Slice the apple thinly and place in a 32-ounce mason jar.

2. Crush the cranberries and place in the jar.

3. Cut the mango flesh off the pit and dice.

4. Place the mango and rosemary in the jar, top up with the water, and chill for 4 hours. Taste to see whether there is a hint of rosemary; if so, remove so it doesn't take over the other flavors.

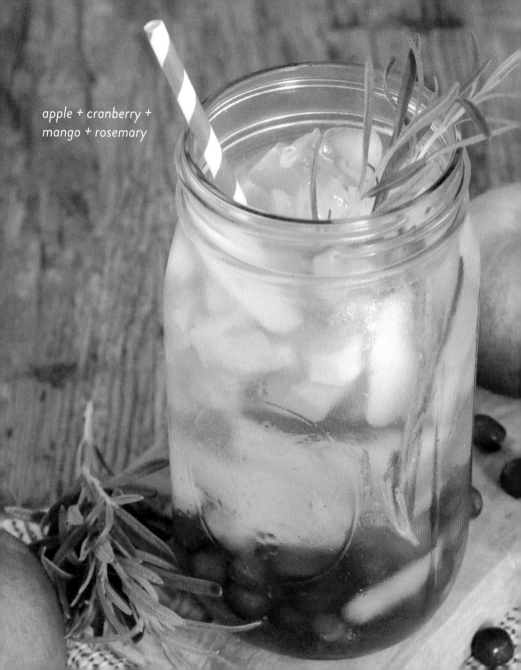

*apple + cranberry +
mango + rosemary*

apple + cinnamon

Apples infuse slowly, so slice them thinly. Remember to eat the apple once the water is infused or before the day is done. Cinnamon is one of the most delicious and healthy spices. It can lower blood sugar levels and reduce the risk of heart attacks, and it has other heart health benefits as well. Cinnamon is an anti-inflammatory and high in antioxidants.

½ apple

1 cinnamon stick

A squeeze of lemon juice

Filtered water

1. Remove the core, seeds, and stem from the apple and slice thinly.

2. Place the apple slices and cinnamon stick in a 32-ounce mason jar, add the lemon juice, and top up with the water.

3. Let chill in the refrigerator for 4 or more hours. Apples take longer to infuse the water, so you can refill the jar after drinking half of the water.

— HEALTH NOTE —

Apples contain phytonutrients, which include many health-promoting properties. Apples are an anti-inflammatory and high in antioxidants. Consuming apples may help reduce the risk of developing hypertension, cancer, heart disease, and diabetes.

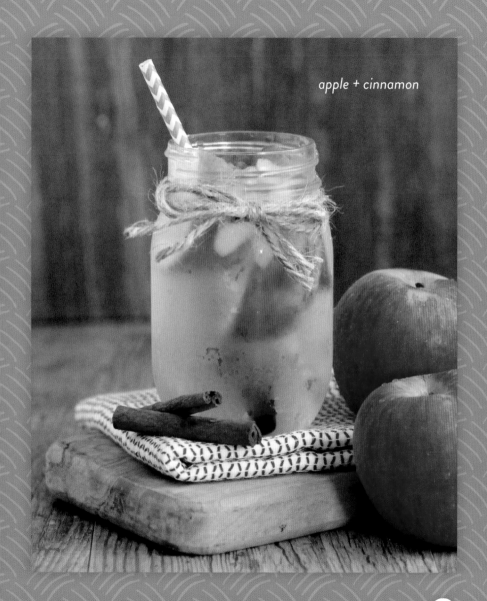

apple + cinnamon

blackberry + kiwi

This beautiful mixture is as tasty as it looks. This pair has a lot in common as well. Both are a good source of vitamin C, which helps digestion and is good for the skin. Eating the fruit will provide many minerals and vitamins as well.

12 blackberries

1 kiwi

Filtered water

1. Cut the blackberries in half.

2. Peel the kiwi if it is not organic and slice into thick slices.

3. Add the blackberries and kiwi to a 32-ounce mason jar and top up with the water. Chill for 4 hours to infuse. Best cold. If there is no time to chill, add ice cubes.

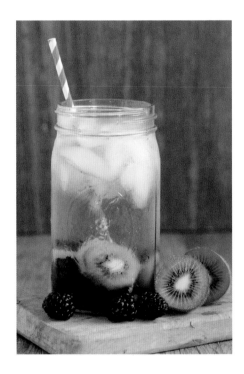

blackberry + mint + lime

Blackberries are truly one of the most beautiful fruits. Their color immediately lets you know they are healthy. Mixing in a little lime and mint really brings out the flavor in the health-packed berry.

12 blackberries

2 or 3 fresh mint leaves

2 or 3 lime slices

Filtered water

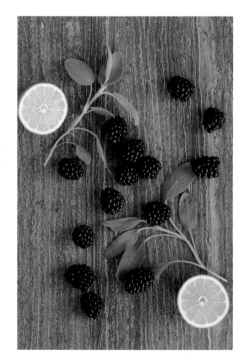

1. Lightly rinse the berries and place in a 32-ounce mason jar.

2. Add the mint and lime slices to the jar and top up with the water. Chill for the best flavor. Remove the rind and white pith of the lime after 4 hours to prevent bitterness.

cucumber + lime + mint

Cucumber makes a light, sweet infusion. Add lime to perk up the drink and a couple mint leaves for that herbal flavor. This is a good drink to have along with meals and goes with just about anything fresh and healthy.

One 3-inch piece cucumber

½ lime

2 fresh mint leaves

Filtered water

1. Peel the cucumber and slice to your desired thickness.

2. Remove the rind and white pith from the lime and slice into rounds.

3. Crush the mint leaves with your fingers.

4. Place the cucumber and lime slices in a jar and add the crushed mint leaves. Top up with the water.

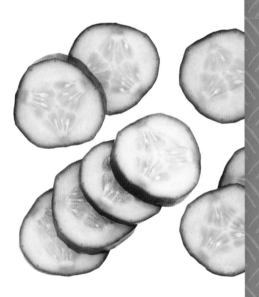

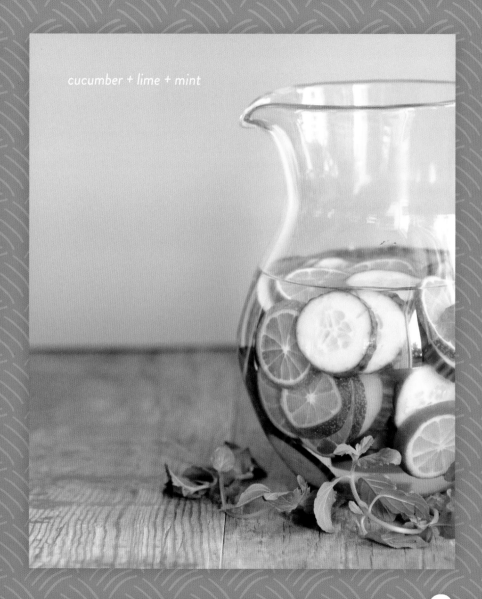

cucumber + lime + mint

honeydew + mint + lime

Honeydew is high in water and potassium, which promotes healthy blood pressure levels. It contains vitamin C and copper, making honeydew good for clear, healthy skin. The cool burst of mint and lime makes this the perfect hydrating drink after a workout.

Enough honeydew
    to make 1 cup

1 sprig mint

1 lime

Filtered water

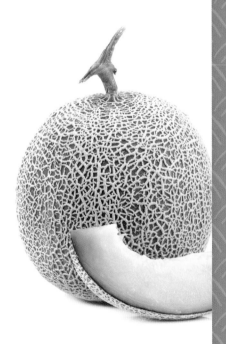

1. Remove the rind from the honeydew and cut the flesh into chunks.

2. Remove the rind and white pith from the lime and slice into rounds.

3. Place the honeydew and lime slices in a 32-ounce mason jar and add the mint. Top up with the water and chill in the refrigerator.

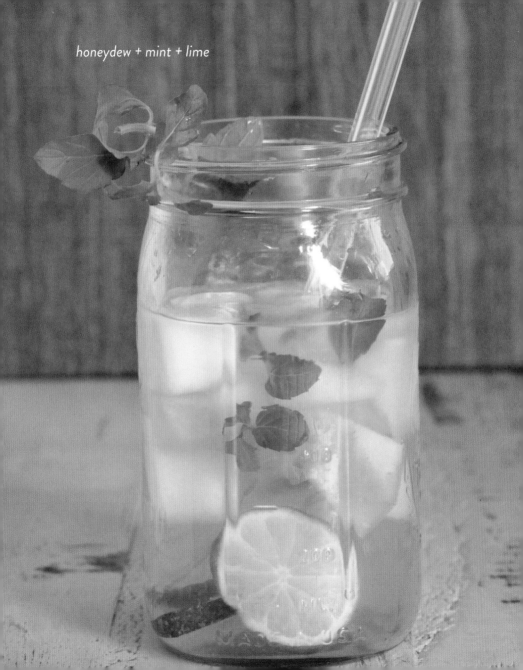

honeydew + mint + lime

kiwi + orange

Kiwi is high in vitamin C and antioxidants and loaded with minerals. It's good for the skin, promotes digestion, and is a source of fiber. Also known for its vitamin C, orange makes a great combination with kiwi for a hydrating, healthy drink.

1 kiwi

½ orange

Filtered water

1. If the kiwi is organic, there is no need to peel off the skin. If the kiwi is inorganic, remove the skin. Slice the kiwi into thick slices.

2. Slice the orange.

3. Place the kiwi and orange slices in a 32-ounce mason jar, top up with the water, and chill for 4 to 6 hours.

4. Eat the fruit throughout the day. Remove the rind and white pith of the orange after 4 hours to prevent bitterness.

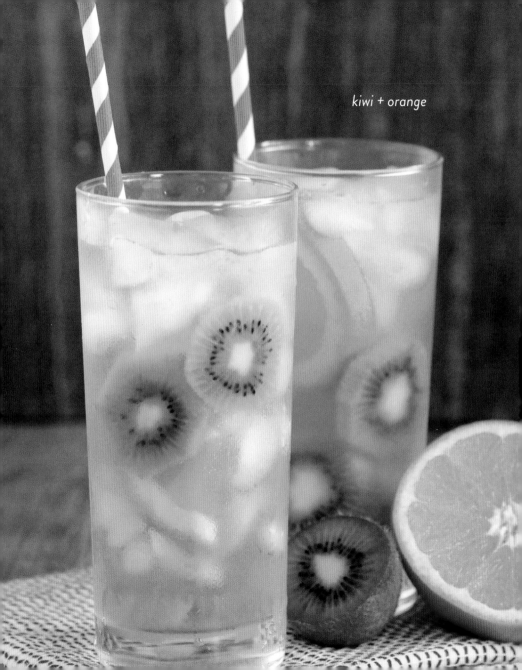

kiwi + orange

lemon + lavender

Culinary lavender has a sweet, floral flavor. It can be purchased online or at a local nursery. It might be seasonal, so when you find some, it's nice to infuse ice cubes to use at another time. Did you know that lavender contains vitamin A, which is good for eye health? Lavender also contains calcium and iron. If you like the taste, go ahead and eat the little buds to obtain the nutrients. If you have extra lavender water at the end of the day, pour it into a hot bath to soak and relax.

3 or 4 lemon slices
1 teaspoon culinary lavender
Filtered water

1. Remove the rind and white pith from the lemon slices. It is best to do this before infusing so as not to overpower and make the lavender bitter.

2. Place the lemon slices and lavender in a 32-ounce mason jar, top up with the water, and chill.

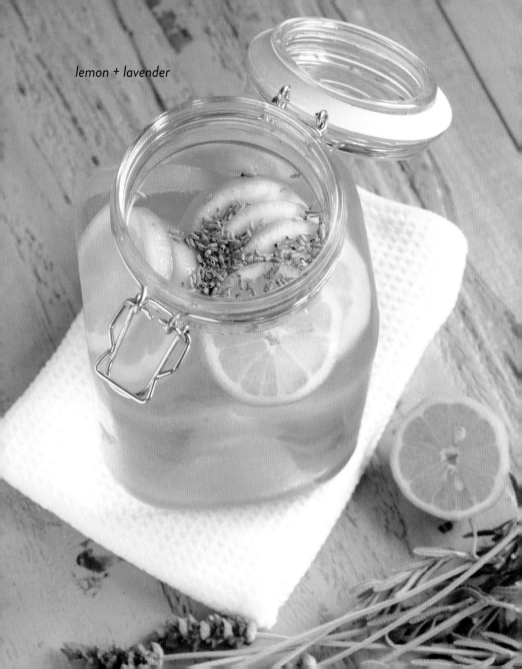

lemon + lavender

lemon + cranberries

Enjoy another beautiful combination with lemon and bright red cranberries in this infusion. For full detoxification benefits, purchase unsweetened cranberry juice and add crushed fresh cranberries.

1 lemon

3 ounces unsweetened cranberry juice

Small handful crushed cranberries

Filtered water

1. Remove the rind and white pith from the lemon and slice.

2. Crush the cranberries on a chopping board with the flat side of a chopping knife. Set the knife on the cranberries and smash the blade firmly with your fist until the cranberries are crushed. Once or twice should be enough.

3. Place the cranberry juice and crushed cranberries in a 32-ounce mason jar.

4. Add the lemon slices, top up the jar with the water, and chill.

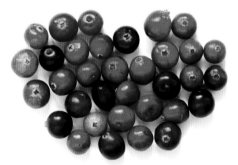

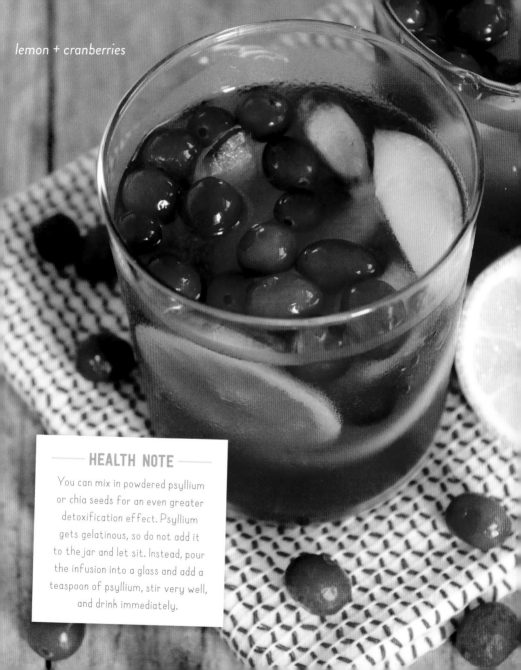

lemon + cranberries

—— HEALTH NOTE ——

You can mix in powdered psyllium
or chia seeds for an even greater
detoxification effect. Psyllium
gets gelatinous, so do not add it
to the jar and let sit. Instead, pour
the infusion into a glass and add a
teaspoon of psyllium, stir very well,
and drink immediately.

lime + ginger

Anticarcinogenic limes and anti-inflammatory ginger are equal stars in this infusion. Ginger can help digestion and fighting colds. To obtain more benefits, the ginger should be crushed.

1 lime

One 1-inch piece fresh ginger

Filtered water

1. Remove the rind and white pith from the lime and slice.

2. To remove the skin from ginger, use a knife or the edge of a teaspoon to scrape off the skin.

3. To crush ginger, make a few cuts in the cut ginger and lay the flat end of a chopping knife on top of the ginger. Use your fist to pound on the knife, which will then crush the ginger.

4. Place the lime slices and ginger in a 32-ounce mason jar and top up with the water.

5. See the note for the Lemon + Crushed Ginger recipe (page 41) for instructions on making ginger tea.

orange +
cinnamon

It's good to include vitamin C in your daily diet, and orange provides this for you. Cinnamon is known to reduce blood sugar and improve concentration.

½ orange
1 cinnamon stick
Filtered water

1. Wash the orange, cut into slices, and remove the rind and white pith, if desired. It's all up to you.

2. Place the orange slices and cinnamon stick in a 32-ounce mason jar, top up with the water, and chill for 4 to 6 hours. If left on, remove the rind and white pith of the orange after 4 hours to prevent bitterness.

3. Put some ice cubes in a glass and pour yourself a mood-lifting infusion.

mango + cucumber + ginger

Mango is high in antioxidants. It can lower cholesterol, clear the skin, improve digestion, and alkalize the body. By eating mango, you will also absorb vitamins A, B6, B2, and C, along with fiber, copper, and vital enzymes. Cucumber and ginger, powerhouses in their own right, add to this tasty drink.

½ mango
One 2-inch piece cucumber
One 1-inch piece fresh ginger
Filtered water

1. Cut the mango off the pit and cube.

2. Peel the cucumber if it is not organic and slice into rounds.

3. Peel the ginger and slice into thin slices.

4. Place the mango, cucumber, and ginger in a 32-ounce mason jar, top up with the water, and chill for 4 or more hours.

5. Mango is a soft fruit, so eat it anytime you feel the water is infused with its flavor. Ginger can also be removed once the water tastes infused with its essence.

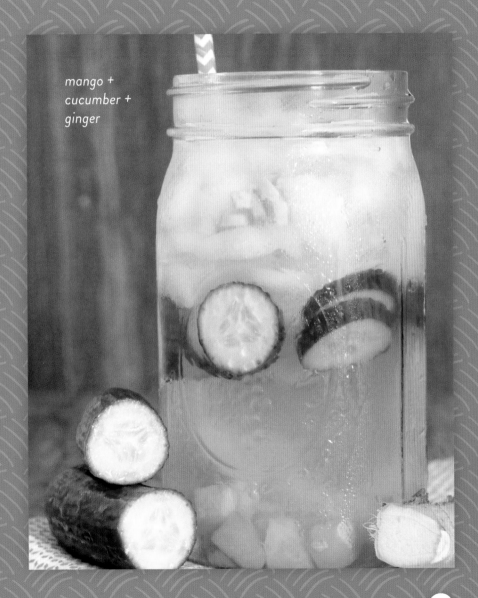

mango +
cucumber +
ginger

peach + basil

Organic summer peaches! Eat them, make pies and ice cream with them, but don't forget to infuse them. Peach infused with basil makes the most delicious summer drink. Crush or muddle the fruit for full flavor and consume the peaches to get all their nutrients. Place ice in a tall glass; pour yourself a refreshing, hydrating drink; and sip away.

1 or 2 peaches

2 or 3 fresh basil leaves

Filtered water

1. Wash the peaches, pit, and slice to your desired thickness or thinness.

2. Place in a 32-ounce mason jar, add the basil, and top up with the water. Chill for 4 hours to infuse. Serve over ice, if desired.

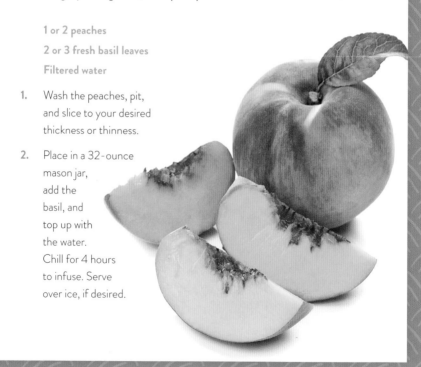

H₂Oh! · Infused Waters for Health and Hydration

pineapple + rosemary + basil

Sweet pineapple and savory herbs make a winning combination. Rosemary is quick to infuse, so remove when the infusion is to your liking. Eating the pineapple will supply you with a multitude of healthy vitamins and nutrients, and will satisfy food cravings as well.

One ½- to ¾-inch-thick slice pineapple

One 1-inch rosemary sprig

2 fresh basil leaves

Filtered water

1. Wash the outer skin of the pineapple slice if you choose to leave it on for the infusion. Cut the pineapple slice into triangle wedges.

2. Rub the rosemary and basil to bruise them slightly and release their essence.

3. Place the pineapple, rosemary, and basil in a 32-ounce mason jar and top up with the water. Let chill in refrigerator for 4 hours.

4. Remove the rosemary when it has infused the water to your liking. Eat the pineapple throughout the day.

raspberry + rosemary + lemon

Raspberries contain vitamin C and magnesium. They have anti-inflammatory properties and help slow the aging process. The added small piece of rosemary and some lemon slices offer you a deliciously hydrating, full-flavored infusion.

½ to 1 cup raspberries

One 1-inch rosemary sprig

2 or 3 lemon slices

Filtered water

1. Raspberries are very delicate, so rinse them lightly and pick out any soft or spoiled ones. Place them and the rosemary in a 32-ounce mason jar.

2. Remove the rind and white pith from the lemon slices and place in the jar.

3. Top up with the water and infuse 4 hours in the refrigerator.

4. Remove the rosemary when water is to your liking. Consume the raspberries throughout the day or as soon as the infusion tastes good to you.

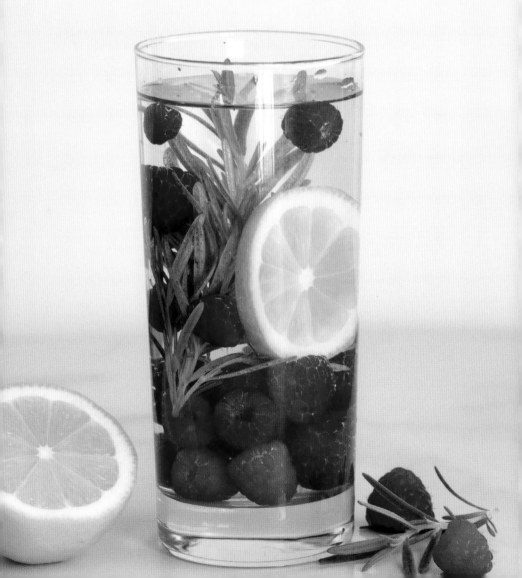

raspberry + rosemary + lemon

strawberry + lemon + rosemary

When strawberries are in season, it's the time to use them for infusions. In this recipe, cut the rinds and white pith off the lemon so as not to overpower the sweetness of the strawberries. If you choose to infuse with the lemon rind on, only leave in for 1 hour. Then cut the rinds off and place the lemon back in the infusion. Rosemary is quite strong, so use only a small piece and taste after a couple of hours.

5 or 6 strawberries
½ lemon
One 1-inch rosemary sprig
Filtered water

1. Wash and hull the strawberries and cut in half.

2. Remove the rind and white pith from the lemon and slice.

3. Place the strawberries, lemon, and rosemary in a 32-ounce mason jar and top up with the water.

4. Infuse for 4 hours and test for taste. After the water is infused with the flavors, you can eat the strawberries for nutritional value and their delicious taste. Strawberries left too long in water soften quickly. Chill or add ice.

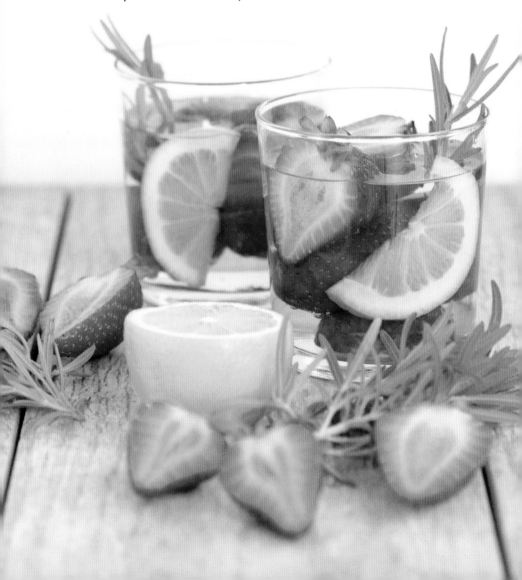

strawberry + lemon + rosemary

strawberry + mint + lime

The potassium in strawberries promotes bone health, and their flavonoids may lower the risk of heart disease. Strawberries infuse the flavor of water quickly, as it's a soft fruit. Taste the water a couple of hours after infusing, and if the flavor suits your taste, eat the strawberries for maximum nutrients. If not quite ready, leave in the strawberries for another hour or so. Mint mixed with strawberry enhances the infusion and is good for digestion. With a hint of lime for vitamin C, you have a delicious, refreshing summer drink.

5 or 6 strawberries

2 or 3 mint leaves

½ lime

Filtered water

1. Wash and hull the strawberries and cut in half.

2. Remove the peel and white pith from the lime and cut into slices.

3. Place the strawberries in a 32-ounce mason jar along with mint and sliced lime. Top up with the water and chill.

— FRESH NOTE —

Be sure to always buy organic strawberries, as conventionally grown strawberries hold the highest amount of pesticides and chemicals from nonorganic growing practices.

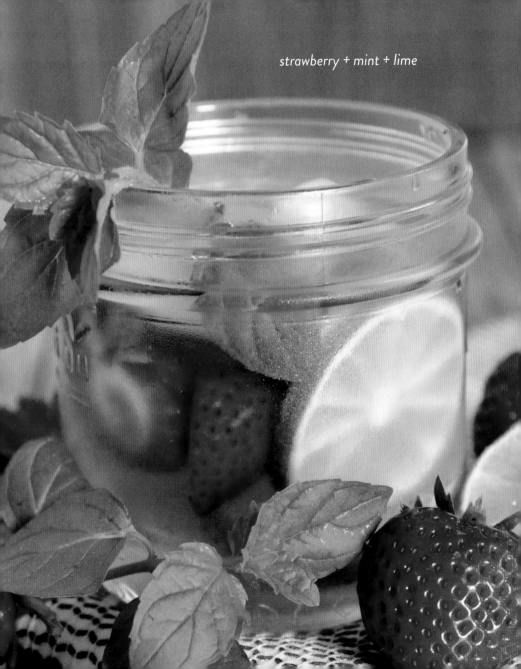

strawberry + mint + lime

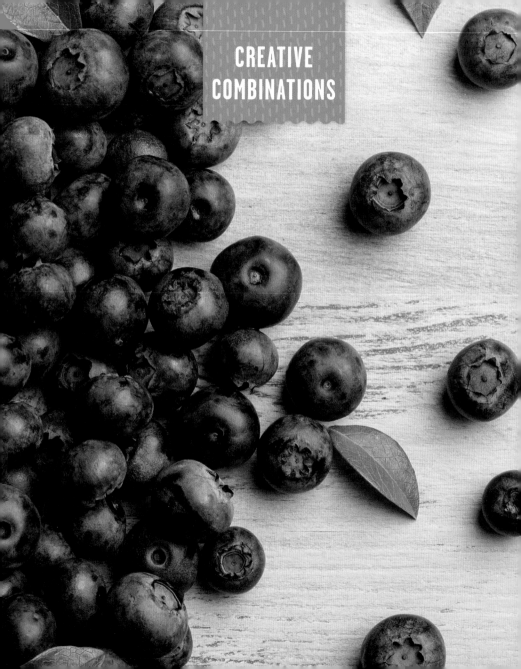

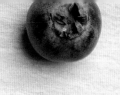

blueberry + cilantro

Consuming blueberries daily as a snack or from your water bottle can make a difference in your antioxidant intake. Blueberries are important to a healthy diet. If you are not a cilantro lover, then it can be replaced in this drink with flat-leaf parsley. Either way, the infusion of blueberries and herb can be eaten for full benefit. It's like having your water and eating it too.

½ to 1 cup blueberries

3 or 4 sprigs cilantro or flat-leaf parsley, with stems

Filtered water

1. Wash the blueberries and place in a 32-ounce mason jar.

2. Add the cilantro, top up with the water, and chill for 4 hours to infuse.

3. Eat the blueberries and cilantro for their full nutritional benefit.

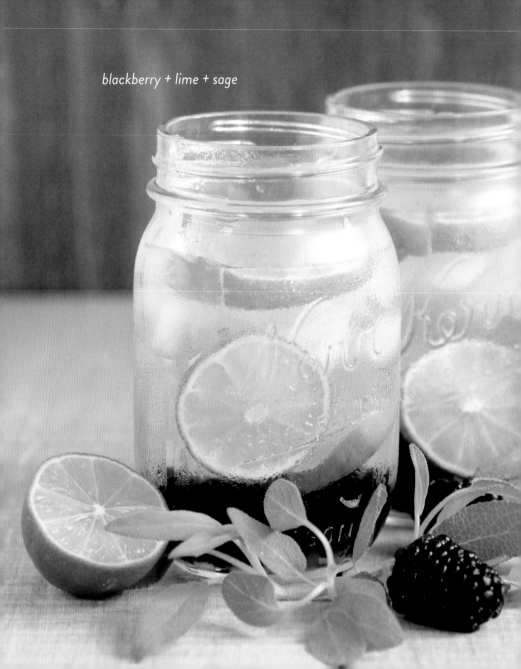

blackberry + lime + sage

blackberry + lime + sage

Your taste buds will be happy with this berry, citrus, herb mixture. Blackberries, which are high in vitamin C, can help keep you healthy. Sage is an amazing herb that can lower inflammation, improve brain function, and regulate digestion. When combined with lime, the result is very tasty and different, in a good way.

12 blackberries

3 or 4 lime slices

4 fresh sage leaves

Filtered water

1. Place the blackberries, limes, and sage that has been lightly crushed in your hand in a 32-ounce mason jar.

2. Top up with the water and chill for 4 or more hours. Remove the rind and white pith of the lime after 4 hours to prevent bitterness.

— HEALTH NOTE —

Sage tea is good for hot flashes, menstrual period, depression, insomnia, memory loss, and digestive issues. Make 2 cups of sage tea by lightly boiling the sage in water. Let steep for 15 or more minutes. Allow the tea to cool and add to the infusion as some of the water. By making a tea, you will extract all the benefits from the leaves.

blueberry + mint + orange

Blueberries are a superfood, meaning their nutritional value is very high. Studies show eating blueberries is helpful for many conditions and areas of the body, including heart, brain, diabetes, blood pressure, cholesterol, and antiaging, to name a few areas of functional support. This infusion combination is a perfect complement of flavors. Eat the blueberries and orange slices for their complete nutritional value.

½ to 1 cup blueberries

2 fresh mint leaves

3 orange slices

Filtered water

1. Wash the blueberries, crush the mint leaves, and place both in a 32-ounce mason jar.

2. Slice the orange and remove the rind and white pith, or leave on for 4 hours while infusing. Place the orange slices in the jar, top up with the water, and chill for 4 hours. If left on, remove the rind and white pith of the orange after 4 hours to prevent bitterness.

3. If you are taking the water to work or the gym, bring along a long-handled spoon so you can eat the blueberries throughout the day.

blueberry + lime

Simple and delicious blueberries and lime is a photo shoot waiting to happen. The colors beckon you to drink the water. Give a little squeeze of the lime into the water for extra zip. Eat the blueberries for full nutritional value. Throw some infused ice cubes in for an extra treat.

½ to 1 cup blueberries

¼ lime juiced

½ lime sliced

Filtered water

1. Place the blueberries, lime juice, and lime slices in a 32-ounce mason jar.

2. Top up with the water and chill for 4 or more hours. Remove the rind and white pith of the lime after 4 hours to prevent bitterness.

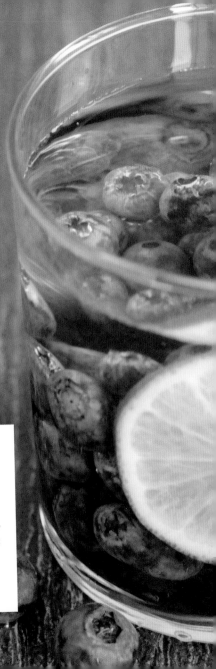

HEALTH NOTE

Eating blueberries daily can supply you with a source of antioxidants and vitamins C and K, and manganese. A full cup is only 84 calories. If you want to infuse with a full cup of blueberries, go right ahead. Blueberries are known to protect against aging and cancer, so be sure to eat all the blueberries along with drinking the water for ultimate nutritional value.

blueberry + orange + basil

With this infusion, you will have all the blueberry benefits and vitamin C from the orange to snack on during the day. It's like a fruit cocktail in a jar. Infuse for 4 hours and eat the orange after that time. Blueberries will stay fresh in the water longer. Eat blueberries and drink throughout the day, which will prevent false hunger pangs. The basil is for flavor, so remove it when the infusion tastes good to you. Basil flavors the water quickly.

½ to 1 cup blueberries

½ orange

2 fresh basil leaves

Filtered water

1. Wash the berries and place them in a 32-ounce mason jar.

2. Slice the orange to desired size and remove the seeds.

3. Crush the basil leaves and add them to the jar along with the orange slices.

4. Top up the jar with the water and chill for 4 hours to infuse.

5. Taste, and remove the basil if the water has picked up the infusion. Eat the orange slices or cut off the rind and white pith and place back in the water for a longer infusion.

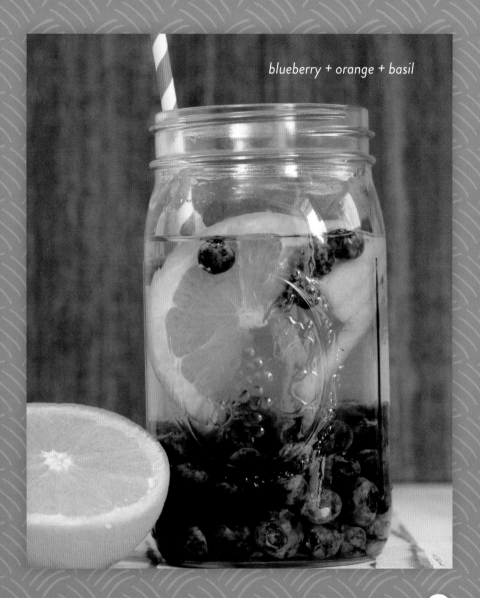

blueberry + orange + basil

blueberry + cucumber + celery

This infusion is so refreshing, it's a perfect thirst quencher. It delivers extra nutrients, as everything can be eaten after the water is well infused. It's like a salad in a jar. Cucumber and celery infuse quite quickly, so check at about 4 hours' time to see whether they have done their job. Blueberries can last much longer, so you might enjoy eating those throughout the day.

½ to 1 cup blueberries
One 2- to 3-inch piece cucumber
1 celery rib
Filtered water

1. Wash the blueberries and place in a 32-ounce mason jar.

2. Peel the cucumber, if you desire, or leave the skin on. Slice and place in a 32-ounce mason jar.

3. Cut the top and bottom off the celery rib and cut the remaining stalk into three pieces. Add the celery to the jar.

4. Top up the jar with the water and chill for 4 or more hours.

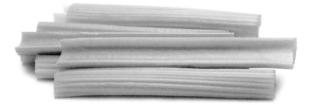

kiwi + cucumber + celery

A kiwi is beautiful, with its bright green flesh and tiny black seeds. No one but Mother Nature could have perfected this beauty. Loaded with antioxidants that are good for digestion and your skin, kiwi contains a multitude of vitamins and minerals. Cucumber is also a skin freshener and thirst quencher. With the addition of celery, which contains a beneficial enzyme and vitamins B6, C, and K, which help improve your blood pressure and cholesterol, this infusion becomes a powerful drink. Eat the kiwi, celery, and cucumber for all their benefits. Enjoy this very refreshing infusion to keep you hydrated all day.

1 kiwi

One 2-inch piece cucumber

1 celery rib

Filtered water

1. Peel the kiwi and cucumber if they are not organic and slice.

2. Cut the celery into two or three pieces.

3. Place the kiwi, cucumber, and celery in a 32-ounce mason jar and top up with the water. Chill for 4 or more hours.

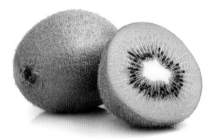

cucumber + jalapeño + mint or cilantro

If you are ready for a little pick-me-up, then this is the infusion for you. The capsaicin contain in the pepper helps burn belly fat and reduces inflammation. We already love cucumber and mint or cilantro, but if you like spice, you will love this infusion.

One 3-inch piece cucumber
½ small jalapeño pepper
2 fresh mint leaves or 3 sprigs cilantro
Filtered water

1. Peel the cucumber, if you desire, or leave the skin on. Slice and place in a 32-ounce mason jar.

2. Remove the seeds from the jalapeño, slice the pepper into rounds, and place in the jar.

3. Add your choice of crushed mint or cilantro, top up with the water, and chill.

4. After the ingredients have infused the water to your liking, you can remove the fruit and continue to drink the water. Refill the water when the jar is half full if the infusion gets too strong.

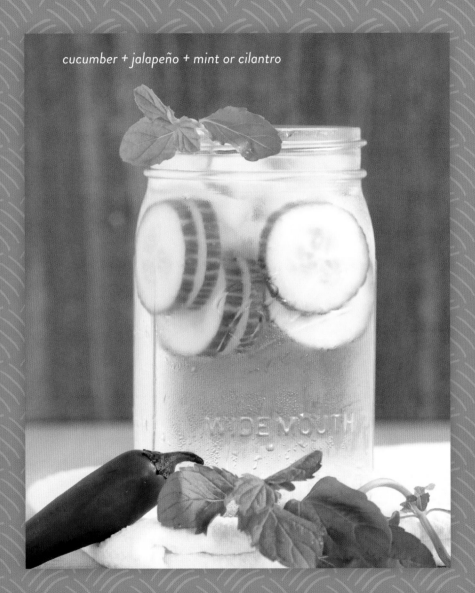

cucumber + jalapeño + mint or cilantro

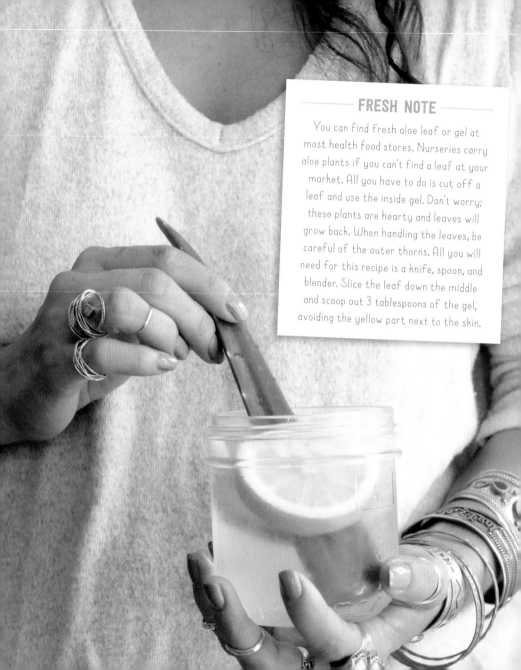

FRESH NOTE

You can find fresh aloe leaf or gel at most health food stores. Nurseries carry aloe plants if you can't find a leaf at your market. All you have to do is cut off a leaf and use the inside gel. Don't worry; these plants are hearty and leaves will grow back. When handling the leaves, be careful of the outer thorns. All you will need for this recipe is a knife, spoon, and blender. Slice the leaf down the middle and scoop out 3 tablespoons of the gel, avoiding the yellow part next to the skin.

lemon + aloe vera

Aloe vera is a green cactus that has many health benefits. It's a type of protein, which contains 20 amino acids, and vitamins A, B, C, and E. Aloe is also antiviral and antibacterial and is especially good for our skin. It can help decrease inflammation and aid in stomach issues.

3 tablespoons aloe gel

4 cups filtered water

1 lemon

A squeeze or two of fresh lemon or orange juice (optional)

1. Place the gel and water in a blender and blitz until smooth.

2. Slice the lemon.

3. Pour the gel mixture into a 32-ounce mason jar and add the lemon slices.

4. Taste and add a squeeze or two of lemon juice. You can also use a squeeze of orange juice, if desired. Chill and drink cold. Remove the rind and white pith of the lemon after 4 hours to prevent bitterness.

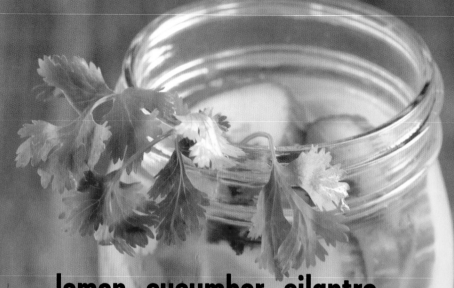

lemon + cucumber + cilantro

This infusion combination is especially hydrating and will refresh you quickly after a workout.

½ lemon

4 sprigs cilantro with stems

One 3-inch piece cucumber

Filtered water

1. Slice the lemon.

2. Gently crush the cilantro to activate its essential oils.

3. Peel the cucumber, if you desire, or leave the skin on. Slice and place in a 32-ounce mason jar.

4. Place the lemon slices, crushed cilantro, and cucumber to the jar and top up with the water.

5. Refrigerate for 4 hours or overnight. Remove the rind and white pith of the lemon after 4 hours to prevent bitterness.

lemon + mint + cucumber + grapefruit

Lemon is a detoxifier and has a delicious citrus taste. Mint is great for digestion and is gently stimulating. Cucumber is effective in ridding the body of toxins. Cut thick slices of grapefruit for the infusion and eat them within for 4 hours to take advantage of the fruit's immunity-boosting and vitamin C benefits.

4 to 8 lemon slices

2 thick slices grapefruit

1 to 3 fresh mint leaves

4 medium-thick slices peeled or unpeeled cucumber

Filtered water

1. Place the lemon and grapefruit slices, mint, and cucumber in a 32-ounce mason jar and top up with the water.

2. Refrigerate 4 hours, taste, and remove the rind and white pith of the lemon and grapefruit to prevent bitterness. If the grapefruit infusion is strong enough for your liking, eat the grapefruit for its complete nutrition. This water can sit in the refrigerator overnight, but remember that citrus rind and pith left in longer than 4 hours can bitter the water.

mango + basil + lime

Mango-infused water tastes great, especially with the addition of basil and lime. Mango is loaded with nutrients and vitamins. Drinking the water and eating the fruit makes for an easy way to get hydrated and obtain vitamins all in one container. You will be filling your jar more than once with these ingredients.

½ mango
3 fresh basil leaves
½ lime
Filtered water

1. Cut the mango off the pit and cube or slice.

2. Slice the lime thinly and place in a 32-ounce mason jar, along with the mango and basil. Top up with the water and chill for 4 or more hours. Remove the rind and white pith of the lime after 4 hours to prevent bitterness.

3. Eat the fruit once the water is infused, or add more water for a second round of hydration.

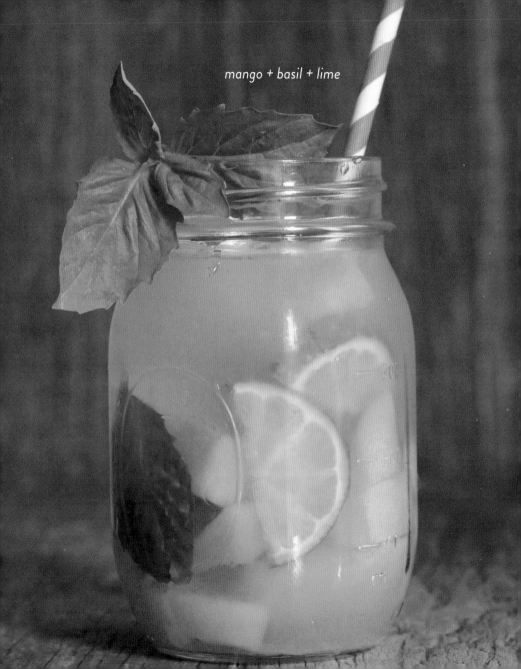

mango + basil + lime

orange + pineapple + mint

This tropical combination will help curb your appetite. Pineapple contains a digestive enzyme and may help with congestion of the lungs. The infusion is for flavor and hydration, and eating the fruit provides its nutrients. Pineapple is good for eye health and bone strength. Pineapple also has anti-inflammatory benefits.

½ orange

One ½- to ¾-inch slice pineapple

2 fresh mint leaves

Filtered water

1. Slice the orange.

2. Crush the mint leaves between your fingers.

3. Wash the outer skin of the pineapple slice if you choose to leave it on for the infusion. Slice the pineapple into triangles and place in a 32-ounce mason jar along with the orange and mint.

4. Top up the jar with the water and refrigerate for 4 hours or more. Remove the rind and white pith of the orange after 4 hours to prevent bitterness. Eat the fruit when the water is infused to your liking. The fruit holds all the nutrition, so enjoy your snack. Eating the fruit helps you meet your daily nutritional requirements.

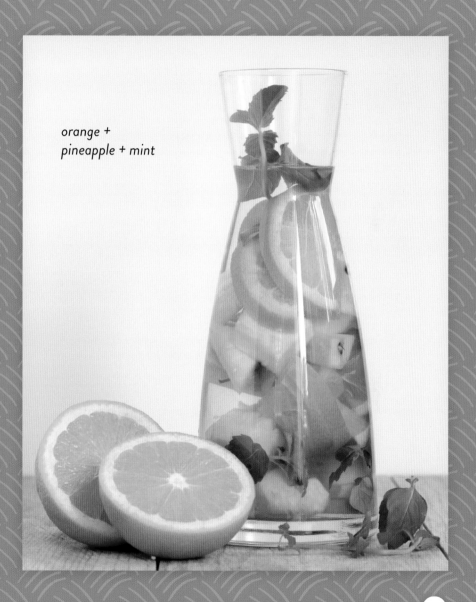

orange +
pineapple + mint

orange + star anise

A beautiful infusion is in store for you. Pairing orange, with its high vitamin C content and sweet taste, with star anise creates a unique flavor. Making star anise tea and using the water in this infusion is the best way to extract the nutritional value of the seed, which contains vitamin C that helps protect the body against cellular damage caused by free radicals. Star anise also has antifungal and antibacterial capabilities. This infusion can assist in alleviating cramps, bloating, and indigestion.

Filtered water

5 star anise

½ orange

1. To make star anise tea, lightly boil 4 cups of the water and shut off the heat. Place the star anise in the pan. Cover and let steep for 15 minutes, or until the flavor is to your liking. Pour into a glass container and chill overnight.

2. Wash the orange and slice. You can remove the rind and white pith or keep it on.

3. Place the orange slices in the jar and top up with the cooled star anise tea. It's delicious well chilled and with ice cubes.

4. Be sure to eat the orange after 4 to 6 hours for its nutritional value, and to remove its rind and white pith after 4 hours if continuing to infuse, to prevent bitterness.

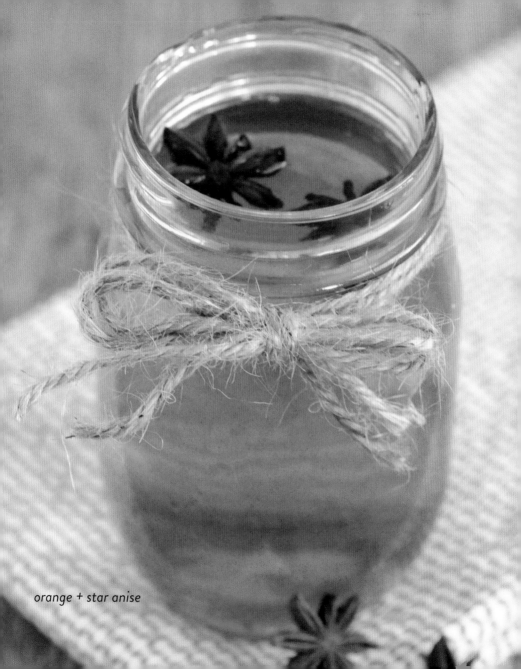

orange + star anise

raspberry + pear + orange

Pep up your day with this infused combination. The beta-carotene in oranges protects your skin. Oranges are packed with vitamin C and good for cancer prevention and high blood pressure. Remember, you have to actually eat the orange to get these benefits. Raspberries are a high–vitamin C berry, so eat the little berries along with your orange slices. The water will be infused and you can enjoy snacking on the fruit. Don't forget to eat the pear slices as well, as they will add to your daily recommended fruit intake. If you don't have a pear, add sliced apple instead.

½ to 1 cup raspberries
¼ or more pear
3 orange slices
Filtered water

1. Lightly wash the raspberries and pick out any damaged or soft ones.

2. Slice the pear into thick slices.

3. Remove the peel and white pith from the orange and slice into rounds.

4. Place all the fruit in a 32-ounce mason jar and top up with the water. Chill for about 4 hours. Remove the rind and white pith of the orange after 4 hours to prevent bitterness.

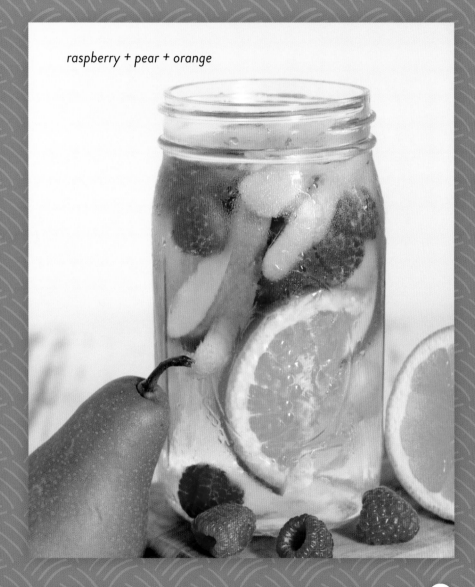

raspberry + pear + orange

watermelon + basil + balsamic vinegar

The tastier the water, the more we drink. The more we drink, the better our health. This combination will spark your desire to consume more water. You've learned the benefits of eating watermelon in our other recipes, and this recipe is no different. Eat the fruit after infusion is complete to obtain all its nutrients. Give it a try!

Several slices watermelon

3 fresh basil leaves

1 teaspoon balsamic vinegar (best quality possible)

Filtered water

1. Cut the watermelon slices into triangles. If using an organic melon, you can leave the rind on.

2. Place the melon, basil, and balsamic vinegar in a 32-ounce mason jar.

3. Top up with the water and give it a shake or stir. Chill for 4 hours and serve over ice, if desired. Basil ice cubes can be added as well (see page 16 for directions).

watermelon +
honeydew + mint

The taste of ripe honeydew is sweet and
satisfying and makes a delicious breakfast.
Use any leftovers for a water infusion to
keep you hydrated all day. Honeydew
contains vitamin C, which is good for your
skin, and potassium, which is good for heart
function. Pair it with watermelon for a
sweet treat and appetite suppressant.

½ cup watermelon chunks

½ cup honeydew chunks

2 fresh mint leaves

Filtered water

1. Cut the melon chunks into your
   desired pieces and remove the rind.

2. Place the melon pieces and mint in a
   32-ounce mason jar and top up with
   the water.

3. Chill for 4 hours in the refrigerator. Fill
   a glass with ice and pour in the infusion
   and some fruit pieces. This will be a
   delicious drink for a break in your day.

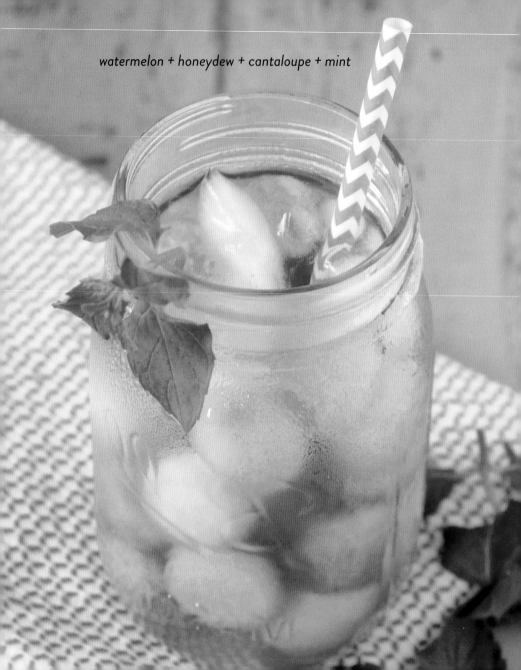

watermelon + honeydew + cantaloupe + mint

watermelon + honeydew + cantaloupe + mint

Infusing water with melon produces a light, sweet taste. This is a beautiful display of summer melons, with lots of nutrition coming from eating the fruit. This infusion is a hydrating drink packed with antioxidants, potassium, vitamin C, and copper.

½ cup watermelon chunks

½ cup honeydew chunks

½ cup cantaloupe chunks

2 to 3 mint leaves

Filtered water

1. Cut melons into desired pieces and remove the rind. Place all the ingredients in a 32-ounce mason jar and top up with water.

2. Chill for 4 hours in the refrigerator. Fill a glass with ice and pour in the infusion, including some fruit pieces.

AFTERWORD

Now you are ready for family and friends, a party, or just a beautiful treat for yourself.

It's been my pleasure to bring you some of my favorite combinations of infused waters and ice cubes.

I hope you've had a chance to feel how water affects your body and your health and have learned the importance of hydration. Hopefully you gained a new respect for water, as we must treat our ocean, streams, rivers, and all water with respect by taking care of our environment and holding companies that pollute our oceans accountable.

For a list of nonprofit organizations that work to help improve water conditions around the world and conserve this most valuable resource, visit the Seametrics blog at www.seametrics.com/blog.

ACKNOWLEDGMENTS

I love my family so much and they always let me test my recipes on them. Thanks to my children: Lisa, Jonas, Mia, and Dan. My grandchildren: Mackenzie, Hannah, Karly, Rocky, Luke, Audrey, Gunner, and my always sweet and beautiful daughter-in-law, Gigi.

Thanks to my longtime partner, Mike, who is always by my side looking out for me, being my right-hand man and my all-purpose boyfriend. You are irreplaceable! My dear friend Victoria Dodge who took the photos in this book, you are just the sweetest person and so talented. I'm grateful for your friendship and your creativity for this book. Big, big thanks to Kari Stuart, the talented Ann Treistman for believing in my writing, and the team at The Countryman Press who worked on making this book look good.

Thanks to my friends who make my life fun and continue to inspire and encourage me: my longtime friend Julie Kavner, for egging me on in all my endeavors for decades; Catrinel, my workshop partner, who makes me laugh at nothing and about everything; Robin Leach, who I love and respect and who always encourages me; and Steve Leach, my foodie guy friend. To my other close friends who believe in me: Susan, Miriam and Jens, Ami and Mark, Corinna, Uli and Keanu, Michael and Eileen, Patricia and Hanns, Diana and Andy, Ron and Jeanette, and all the B-Day Girls.

INDEX

H2Oh! · Infused Waters for Health and Hydration